Meningioma - The Essentials from Bench to Bedside

Edited by Sara Hanaei and Seyed Farzad Maroufi

Published in London, United Kingdom

Meningioma - The Essentials from Bench to Bedside
http://dx.doi.org/10.5772/intechopen.1000388
Edited by Sara Hanaei and Seyed Farzad Maroufi

Contributors
Amit Kumar Chowhan, Catalina Rojas-Solé, Claudio Lühr, Dongxia Feng, Farnam Mohebi, Fateme Montazeri, Francisco Bova, Frank Y. Shan, Gonzalo Miranda, Gustavo Zomosa, Hamidreza Komaki, Hannaneh Kabir, Jason H. Huang, Jennifer H. Murillo, José Lorenzoni, Karming Fung, Lene Troncoso, Lucas González-Johnson, Mohsen Merati, Mousmi Agrawal, Sara Hanaei, Seyed Farzad Maroufi, Yilu Zhang

First published in London, United Kingdom, 2024 by IntechOpen
IntechOpen is the global imprint of INTECHOPEN LIMITED, registered in England and Wales, registration number: 11086078, 167-169 Great Portland Street, London, W1W 5PF, United Kingdom

British Library Cataloguing-in-Publication Data
A catalogue record for this book is available from the British Library

Additional hard and PDF copies can be obtained from orders@intechopen.com

Meningioma - The Essentials from Bench to Bedside
Edited by Sara Hanaei and Seyed Farzad Maroufi
p. cm.
Print ISBN 978-0-85466-146-6
Online ISBN 978-0-85466-145-9
eBook (PDF) ISBN 978-0-85466-147-3

For EU product safety concerns:
IN TECH d.o.o., Prolaz Marije Krucifikse Kozulić 3, 51000 Rijeka, Croatia,
info@intechopen.com or visit our website at intechopen.com.

Meet the editors

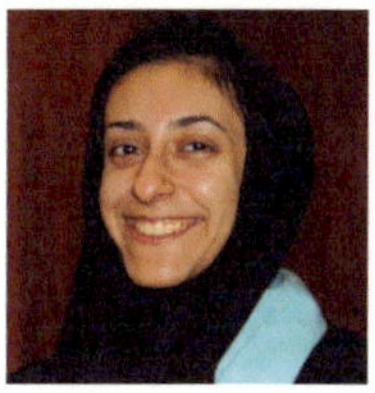

Dr. Sara Hanaei started medicine at TUMS in 2010 and received a Master of public health (MPH) degree in 2014. She graduated with MD-MPH in 2018. She also received a TUMS research diploma (TUMS-RD) in a two-year study period from 2013 to 2015. She was a research assistant at the Research Center for Immunodeficiencies (RCID) from 2018 to 2021 and further continued neurosurgery as a clinical specialty at TUMS in 2021. She has experience in teaching research skills to students. Medical research was one of her greatest interests since the beginning of her academic education, especially in neurosurgery and immunology; therefore, she started research in those fields. Over the past decade, she has contributed to different research projects, books, and other research activities including instructing research workshops in statistics, systematic reviews, and meta-analysis. She got involved in executive tasks and developed some executive skills through membership in the Universal Scientific Education and Research Network (USERN), where she experienced organizing scientific events, congresses, festivals, scoring, rankings, and so forth. She co-edited a two-volume book:

- Human Brain and Spinal Cord Tumors: From Bench to Bedside. Volume 1 (Neuroimmunology and Neurogenetics)
- Human Brain and Spinal Cord Tumors: From Bench to Bedside. Volume 2 (The Path to Bedside Management).

In early 2024, she co-founded Borderless Research, Advancement, and Innovation in Neuroscience Network (BRAINet), which was intended to serve in a multidisciplinary and cross-disciplinary manner and embrace all aspects of neuroscience. On this account, different disciplines in neuroscience may come together in the BRAINet, including theoretical and molecular neuroscience, clinical neuroscience (neurology), surgical neuroscience (neurosurgery), and social neuroscience. In light of the borderless collaboration of seniors and juniors, it is provided to promote scientific activities and step forward to advancement and innovation in neuroscience.

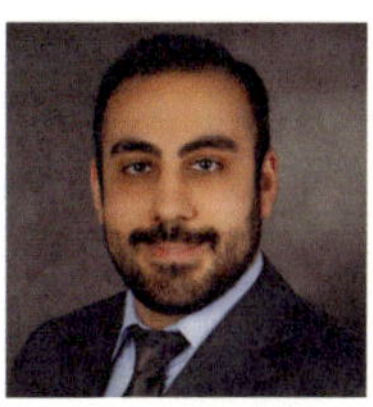

Dr. Farzad Maroufi started his medical training at Tehran University of Medical Sciences. He acquired two masters (master of professional health education and master of public health) during his medical training. He has been a research assistant at the Department of Neurosurgery at Children's Medical Center. He has published more than 60 papers in the field of neurosurgery. He has served as the post-hoc reviewer for several neurosurgery journals. Recently, he co-founded the Neurosurgical Research Network and serves as the managing director of the network, aimed at training researchers and delivering high-quality research in the field. His main field of work focuses on radiosurgery for various brain and spinal lesions.

Contents

Preface

It is with great pleasure that we present this comprehensive volume, *Meningioma – The Essentials from Bench to Bedside*, an anthology dedicated to the multifaceted exploration of meningiomas. This book aims to bridge the gap between fundamental research and clinical practice in the study of meningiomas, offering readers an in-depth exploration of the multifaceted aspects of this prevalent central nervous system tumor.

Meningiomas are a diverse group of tumors arising from the meninges, the membranous layers surrounding the brain and spinal cord. Despite being typically benign, these tumors can present significant clinical challenges due to their location, size, and potential for recurrence. The intricate nature of meningiomas necessitates a multidisciplinary approach to understanding their pathology, diagnosis, treatment, and the quality of life of affected patients. This volume endeavors to provide a holistic overview, from molecular insights to therapeutic strategies, thus serving as a valuable resource for both researchers and clinicians.

The book is organized into five comprehensive chapters, each delving into critical aspects of meningioma research and management. After the introductory chapter, the second chapter, "Diagnosis and Grading of Meningiomas", provides a foundational understanding of the molecular and genetic underpinnings of meningiomas. It discusses the latest advancements in the molecular characterization of these tumors, shedding light on the genetic mutations and alterations that drive their development. This chapter also covers diagnostic techniques, including imaging modalities and biopsy methods, that are pivotal for accurate identification and classification of meningiomas.

Following this, chapter 3, titled "Quality of Life in Patients with Meningioma" shifts the focus to the patient experience. This chapter addresses the physical, emotional, and cognitive impacts of meningiomas and their treatments. It highlights the importance of considering quality-of-life outcomes in clinical decision-making and provides valuable insights into patient-centered care practices. The chapter emphasizes the necessity of a holistic approach to treatment that goes beyond mere tumor control, advocating for interventions that enhance the overall well-being of patients.

Chapter 4, "Radiosurgery for Intracranial Meningiomas" explores one of the most advanced therapeutic options available for the treatment of these tumors. Radiosurgery has emerged as a critical tool in the management of meningiomas, offering a minimally invasive alternative to traditional surgical techniques. This chapter discusses the principles of radiosurgery, patient selection criteria, and the efficacy and safety profiles of various radiosurgical techniques. It also reviews recent technological advancements that have improved the precision and outcomes of radiosurgical treatments.

The final chapter, "Molecular Alterations, Histopathology and Squash Cytology of Meningioma" delves deeper into the pathological and cytological aspects of meningiomas. It provides an exhaustive review of the histopathological features that distinguish different subtypes of meningiomas and the molecular alterations that are characteristic of these tumors. The chapter also introduces squash cytology as a rapid and effective intraoperative diagnostic technique, highlighting its role in guiding surgical decision-making and improving patient outcomes.

This volume is the result of the collaborative efforts of numerous experts who have contributed their knowledge and expertise. We extend our heartfelt gratitude to all the authors and reviewers for their invaluable contributions. Special thanks go to all the authors for their exceptional contributions and commitment to this project.

We hope that *Meningioma – The Essentials from Bench to Bedside* will serve as a definitive reference for both seasoned professionals and those new to the field, inspiring further research and advancing the understanding and management of meningiomas.

Sara Hanaei MD, MPH
Department of Neurosurgery,
Imam Khomeini Hospital Complex (IKHC),
Tehran University of Medical Sciences (TUMS),
Tehran, Iran

Borderless Research,
Advancement and Innovation in Neuroscience Network (BRAINet),
Tehran, Iran

Seyed Farzad Maroufi MD, MPH, MPHE
Neurosurgical Research Network (NRN),
Universal Scientific Education and Research Network (USERN),
Tehran, Iran

Department of Neurosurgery,
Tehran University of Medical Sciences,
Tehran, Iran

Chapter 1

Introductory Chapter: Meningioma – The Essentials from Bench to Bedside

Seyed Farzad Maroufi and Sara Hanaei

1. Introduction

Meningiomas arising from the meningeal layers are the most prevalent primary central nervous system (CNS) tumors [1]. These lesions comprise more than 35% of CNS tumors and present a complex and enigmatic challenge in the field of neurosurgery. These tumors are characterized by their slow growth, variable clinical manifestations, and intricate histopathological features. First identified by Rudolf Virchow in the nineteenth century, meningiomas have since been the subject of extensive research and clinical scrutiny, leading to a deeper understanding of their biology, classification, and therapeutic approaches [2].

2. Epidemiology

Meningiomas constitute a substantial portion of primary brain tumors, accounting for approximately 36% of all cases [3]. The incidence of meningiomas is reported to be 1.8 to 13 per 100,000 persons per year, with more than 170,000 affected individuals in the United States [4, 5]. Although they can occur at any age, meningiomas are most frequently diagnosed in older individuals, with a median age of 66 at diagnosis [1, 6, 7]. Meningiomas occurrence has demonstrated a predilection for females as they are affected nearly twice as often as males [1]. It should be noted that this gender predilection observed in meningioma incidence has been shown to be age-dependent, as the rates are more comparable in younger ages. The reasons behind the female predominance remain an area of investigation, with hormonal influences and genetic factors being considered as potential contributors. Despite the predominance of sporadic cases, familial predisposition has been identified in a subset of meningiomas [8].

3. Etiology and risk factors

The etiology of meningiomas, though not fully elucidated, represents a complex interplay of genetic, hormonal, and environmental factors. While the majority of meningiomas are sporadic, emerging evidence points to specific genetic mutations and hereditary syndromes that contribute to their development. Investigating the etiological underpinnings of meningiomas is vital for unraveling the molecular mechanisms driving tumorigenesis and guiding targeted therapeutic interventions.

IntechOpen

Regarding genetic predisposition to meningiomas, chromosomal instability emerges as a prominent molecular hallmark influencing tumor recurrence and prognosis in meningiomas [8–11]. Higher-grade meningiomas, including atypical and anaplastic subtypes, exhibit a more complex cytogenetic profile compared to benign tumors [12–14]. Sporadic high-grade meningiomas and low-grade tumors progressing to higher grades typically demonstrate a higher number of cytogenetic aberrations, which strongly correlates with the risk of recurrence [12–15]. Notably, loss of chromosome 22q, housing the NF2 gene (a tumor suppressor gene), is the most common chromosomal abnormality, occurring in a good proportion of meningiomas and increasing with tumor grade [13, 16]. Overall, the evolving malignant biology of meningiomas correlates with increasing chromosomal and genomic abnormalities, underscoring the need for further research into specific mutations to elucidate key tumorigenic events.

Several familial syndromes are associated with an increased risk of meningiomas, shedding light on the genetic underpinnings of these tumors. Neurofibromatosis Type 2 (NF2), as mentioned earlier, has been found to have a strong association with meningioma development. The result of germline mutations of the NF2 gene has been associated with over 50% of patients developing intracranial meningiomas, often earlier in life and more aggressively than sporadic cases [9, 17, 18]. Gorlin Syndrome, associated with mutations in PTCH1, PTCH2, and SUFU genes, increases meningioma risk due to abnormal signaling in the sonic hedgehog pathway [9, 19]. Cowden Syndrome, part of the PTEN (Phosphatase and tensin homolog) hamartoma tumor syndrome (PHTS), results from PTEN mutations and is linked to an 8.25% incidence of meningiomas [19]. Werner Syndrome, an autosomal recessive disorder, significantly elevates meningioma risk due to dysfunctional WRN gene mutations [20]. BAP1 Tumor Predisposition Syndrome, arising from BAP1 mutations, particularly predisposes individuals to aggressive meningiomas [21]. Familial syndromes associated with SMARCB1 and SMARCE1 mutations, impacting the SWI/SNF chromatin remodeling complex, contribute to familial meningiomatosis, with specific mutations correlating with distinct clinical presentations [22]. Additionally, other syndromes such as Gardener, Li-Fraumeni, Turcot, Rubinstein–Taybi syndrome, von Hippel-Lindau, and multiple endocrine neoplasia type I have been related to the development of meningiomas.

Hormonal influences, particularly estrogen and progesterone, have long been implicated in the development and progression of meningiomas. Studies have shown that meningioma cells often express estrogen and progesterone receptors, suggesting a potential role for these hormones in promoting tumor growth [6]. The observed gender disparity in meningioma incidence, with a higher prevalence in females, further supports the hormonal influence hypothesis. Recent scholars have revealed that the fluctuating hormonal levels during pregnancy and menopause may contribute to the growth of meningiomas [23]. The increased prevalence and growth of meningiomas during reproductive years suggest a potential link between hormonal changes and tumor progression. However, the precise mechanisms by which hormones exert their effects on meningioma cells remain an active area of investigation.

While genetic and hormonal factors play prominent roles in meningioma development, the majority of cases are sporadic. Environmental factors, most importantly radiation exposure, have been associated with an increased risk of meningiomas [8, 24]. Individuals exposed to radiation, either through therapeutic interventions or occupational settings, may exhibit a higher incidence of meningiomas. However, the overall contribution of environmental factors to sporadic meningioma cases remains a subject of ongoing research.

4. Clinical features and pathology

Meningiomas exhibit varied distribution, with common locations being the convexity, parasagittal, spinal, skull base, frontobasal, and sphenoid regions. Grade I tumors tend to occur at the skull base, while higher grades are more prevalent at the convexity, parasagittal, falcine, torcular, and intraventricular regions [22, 25–27].

The clinical presentation of meningiomas is diverse, ranging from asymptomatic incidental findings to severe neurological deficits [17]. The symptoms of meningiomas are primarily determined by their location and size, with tumors in various regions resulting in a distinct manifestation [28]. Accordingly, intracranial meningiomas commonly present with symptoms related to increased intracranial pressure, such as headaches, nausea, and vomiting [28]. Additionally, focal neurological deficits, seizures, and cognitive impairment may occur, depending on the specific brain regions affected by the tumor. Meningiomas arising from the skull base can manifest with symptoms related to cranial nerve involvement, including visual disturbances, facial numbness, and hearing loss [29, 30]. Spinal meningiomas, though less common, can lead to back pain, radiculopathy, and motor or sensory deficits corresponding to the level of spinal cord involvement [30]. Understanding the diverse clinical presentations is crucial for early detection and timely intervention, optimizing the chances of successful treatment.

The World Health Organization (WHO) classification system categorizes meningiomas into three grades based on their histopathological characteristics, providing valuable insights into their clinical behavior and guiding therapeutic decisions [31].

- Grade I: Representing the majority of cases (around 80–90%), Grade I meningiomas are classified as benign tumors. These tumors typically exhibit slow growth and well-defined borders, making them good candidates for resection with a favorable prognosis. This grade consists of various histopathological subtypes, including Meningothelial, Fibrous, Transitional, Psammomatous, and Angiomatous subtypes.

- Grade II Meningiomas (Atypical Meningiomas): Representing a smaller subset of cases (17%), Grade II meningiomas are characterized by more aggressive features, such as increased mitotic activity and a higher likelihood of recurrence. These tumors pose challenges in terms of management and necessitate a more comprehensive treatment approach. This grade consists of various histopathological subtypes, including Chordoid, Clear Cell, and Atypical subtypes.

- Grade III Meningiomas (Anaplastic Meningiomas): Grade III meningiomas, representing the most malignant subtype with poor prognosis (1.7% of all meningiomas), are characterized by marked cellular atypia, high mitotic activity, and increased vascularity. This grade consists of various histopathological subtypes, including Papillary, Rhabdoid, and Anaplastic subtypes.

5. Diagnosis

Accurate diagnosis of meningiomas relies on a combination of clinical evaluation, neuroimaging studies, and histopathological examination. Magnetic resonance imaging (MRI) is the modality of choice for the assessment of meningiomas, providing detailed information about the tumor's location, size, and relationship to surrounding structures. On MRI, meningiomas typically appear as well-circumscribed, dural-based, enhancing masses with variable signal intensity on different sequences [31, 32]. Dural tails found on post-contrast imaging of 70% of meningiomas may assist in differentiating these lesions from other extra-axial tumors [32, 33]. Contrast-enhanced computed tomography (CT) scans may also be employed to assess bony involvement and calcifications within the tumor. In addition, cerebral angiography can aid in evaluating the vascular supply to the tumor, particularly in cases where preoperative embolization is considered to reduce intraoperative blood loss [34].

Histopathological examination of biopsy or surgically resected specimens is essential for verification of the diagnosis and determining the tumor grade [35, 36]. Moreover, immunohistochemistry plays a crucial role in differentiating meningiomas from other CNS neoplasms and identifying specific histological subtypes.

6. Treatment

The therapeutic approach to meningiomas is guided by several factors, including tumor size, location, histological grade, patient age, and comorbidities, as well as the presence of symptoms and neurological deficits. Treatment modalities for meningiomas include observation, surgical resection, radiation therapy, and, rarely, systemic therapy.

Observation with serial neuroimaging may be appropriate for asymptomatic, small (<3 cm), and indolent meningiomas, particularly in elderly patients or those with significant comorbidities [37, 38]. Meanwhile, surgical resection remains the treatment of choice for symptomatic, enlarging, or high-grade meningiomas, aiming for maximal safe resection while preserving neurological function and minimizing morbidity [29, 38]. Achieving gross total resection has been associated with a cure in 70–80% of patients [39].

Radiation therapy, including stereotactic radiosurgery (SRS) and fractionated radiotherapy, has been utilized as the primary treatment option for unresectable lesions [35, 38]. Moreover, radiation-based treatments have a mainstay role in the management of residual or recurrent meningiomas. Adjuvant and salvage radiation therapy is reserved for atypical or malignant meningiomas, high-risk histological subtypes, and incompletely resected tumors to improve local control and delay tumor progression [35, 38].

Salvage systemic therapies, including chemotherapy and targeted molecular agents, are used in the treatment of refractory meningiomas [35, 38]. Regardless, limited evidence is available on their efficacy, and no recommendation is given on their use.

Author details

Seyed Farzad Maroufi[1,2] and Sara Hanaei[3,4*]

1 Neurosurgical Research Network (NRN), Universal Scientific Education and Research Network (USERN), Tehran, Iran

2 Department of Neurosurgery, Tehran University of Medical Sciences, Tehran, Iran

3 Department of Neurosurgery, Imam Khomeini Hospital Complex (IKHC), Tehran University of Medical Sciences (TUMS), Tehran, Iran

4 Borderless Research, Advancement and Innovation in Neuroscience Network (BRAINet), Tehran, Iran

*Address all correspondence to: sara.hanaei@gmail.com

References

[1] Ostrom QT, Cioffi G, Gittleman H, Patil N, Waite K, Kruchko C, et al. CBTRUS statistical report: Primary brain and other central nervous system tumors diagnosed in the United States in 2012-2016. Neuro-Oncology. 2019;**21**(Suppl. 5):v1-v100

[2] Barthélemy EJ, Sarkiss CA, Lee J, Shrivastava RK. The historical origin of the term "meningioma" and the rise of nationalistic neurosurgery. Journal of Neurosurgery JNS. 2016;**125**(5):1283-1290

[3] Shibuya M. Pathology and molecular genetics of meningioma: Recent advances. Neurologia Medico-Chirurgica. 2015;**55**(1):14-27

[4] de Robles P, Fiest KM, Frolkis AD, Pringsheim T, Atta C, St. Germaine-Smith C, et al. The worldwide incidence and prevalence of primary brain tumors: A systematic review and meta-analysis. Neuro-Oncology. 2015;**17**(6):776-783

[5] Buerki RA, Horbinski CM, Kruser T, Horowitz PM, James CD, Lukas RV. An overview of meningiomas. Future Oncology (London, England). 2018;**14**(21):2161-2177

[6] Connolly ID, Cole T, Veeravagu A, Popat R, Ratliff J, Li G. Craniotomy for resection of meningioma: An age-stratified analysis of the MarketScan longitudinal database. World Neurosurgery. 2015;**84**(6):1864-1870

[7] Hortobágyi T, Bencze J, Varkoly G, Kouhsari MC, Klekner Á. Meningioma recurrence. Open Medicine (Warsaw, Poland). 2016;**11**(1):168-173

[8] Wiemels J, Wrensch M, Claus EB. Epidemiology and etiology of meningioma. Journal of Neuro-Oncology. 2010;**99**(3):307-314

[9] Lee YS, Lee YS. Molecular characteristics of meningiomas. Journal of Pathology and Translational Medicine. 2020;**54**(1):45-63

[10] Aizer AA, Abedalthagafi M, Bi WL, Horvath MC, Arvold ND, Al-Mefty O, et al. A prognostic cytogenetic scoring system to guide the adjuvant management of patients with atypical meningioma. Neuro-Oncology. 2016;**18**(2):269-274

[11] Nassiri F, Mamatjan Y, Suppiah S, Badhiwala JH, Mansouri S, Karimi S, et al. DNA methylation profiling to predict recurrence risk in meningioma: Development and validation of a nomogram to optimize clinical management. Neuro-Oncology. 2019;**21**(7):901-910

[12] Lamszus K. Meningioma pathology, genetics, and biology. Journal of Neuropathology and Experimental Neurology. 2004;**63**(4):275-286

[13] Clark VE, Erson-Omay EZ, Serin A, Yin J, Cotney J, Ozduman K, et al. Genomic analysis of non-NF2 meningiomas reveals mutations in TRAF7, KLF4, AKT1, and SMO. Science (New York, N.Y.). 2013;**339**(6123):1077-1080

[14] Al-Rashed M, Foshay K, Abedalthagafi M. Recent advances in meningioma immunogenetics. Frontiers in Oncology. 2019;**9**:1472

[15] Al-Mefty O, Kadri PA, Pravdenkova S, Sawyer JR, Stangeby C, Husain M. Malignant progression in meningioma: Documentation of a

series and analysis of cytogenetic findings. Journal of Neurosurgery. 2004;**101**(2):210-218

[16] Karsy M, Azab MA, Abou-Al-Shaar H, Guan J, Eli I, Jensen RL, et al. Clinical potential of meningioma genomic insights: A practical review for neurosurgeons. Neurosurgical Focus. 2018;**44**(6):E10

[17] Wang N, Osswald M. Meningiomas: Overview and new directions in therapy. Seminars in Neurology. 2018;**38**(1):112-120

[18] Smith MJ, Higgs JE, Bowers NL, Halliday D, Paterson J, Gillespie J, et al. Cranial meningiomas in 411 neurofibromatosis type 2 (NF2) patients with proven gene mutations: Clear positional effect of mutations, but absence of female severity effect on age at onset. Journal of Medical Genetics. 2011;**48**(4):261-265

[19] Kerr K, Qualmann K, Esquenazi Y, Hagan J, Kim DH. Familial syndromes involving Meningiomas provide mechanistic insight into sporadic disease. Neurosurgery. 2018;**83**(6):1107-1118

[20] Lauper JM, Krause A, Vaughan TL, Monnat RJ Jr. Spectrum and risk of neoplasia in Werner syndrome: A systematic review. PLoS One. 2013;**8**(4):e59709

[21] Shankar GM, Santagata S. BAP1 mutations in high-grade meningioma: Implications for patient care. Neuro-Oncology. 2017;**19**(11):1447-1456

[22] Pereira BJA, Oba-Shinjo SM, de Almeida AN, Marie SKN. Molecular alterations in meningiomas: Literature review. Clinical Neurology and Neurosurgery. 2019;**176**:89-96

[23] Gurcay AG, Bozkurt I, Senturk S, Kazanci A, Gurcan O, Turkoglu OF, et al. Diagnosis, treatment, and management strategy of meningioma during pregnancy. Asian Journal of Neurosurgery. 2018;**13**(1):86-89

[24] al-Mefty O, Kersh JE, Routh A, Smith RR. The long-term side effects of radiation therapy for benign brain tumors in adults. Journal of Neurosurgery. 1990;**73**(4):502-512

[25] Huntoon K, Toland AMS, Dahiya S. Meningioma: A review of Clinicopathological and molecular aspects. Frontiers in Oncology. 2020;**10**:579599

[26] Magill ST, Young JS, Chae R, Aghi MK, Theodosopoulos PV, McDermott MW. Relationship between tumor location, size, and WHO grade in meningioma. Neurosurgical Focus. 2018;**44**(4):E4

[27] Voß KM, Spille DC, Sauerland C, Suero Molina E, Brokinkel C, Paulus W, et al. The Simpson grading in meningioma surgery: Does the tumor location influence the prognostic value? Journal of Neuro-oncology. 2017;**133**(3):641-651

[28] Meling TR, Da Broi M, Scheie D, Helseth E. Meningiomas: skull base versus non-skull base. Neurosurgical Review. 2019;**42**(1):163-173

[29] Marosi C, Hassler M, Roessler K, Reni M, Sant M, Mazza E, et al. Meningioma. Critical Reviews in Oncology/hematology. 2008;**67**(2):153-171

[30] Whittle IR, Smith C, Navoo P, Collie D. Meningiomas. Lancet (London, England). 2004;**363**(9420):1535-1543

[31] Louis DN, Perry A, Wesseling P, Brat DJ, Cree IA, Figarella-Branger D, et al. The 2021 WHO classification

of tumors of the central nervous system: A summary. Neuro-Oncology. 2021;**23**(8):1231-1251

[32] Huang RY, Bi WL, Griffith B, Kaufmann TJ, la Fougère C, Schmidt NO, et al. Imaging and diagnostic advances for intracranial meningiomas. Neuro-Oncology. 2019;**21**(Suppl. 1):i44-i61

[33] Sotiriadis C, Vo QD, Ciarpaglini R, Hoogewoud HM. Cystic meningioma: Diagnostic difficulties and utility of MRI in diagnosis and management. BMJ Case Reports. 26 Mar 2015;**2015**:bcr2014208274. DOI: 10.1136/bcr-2014-208274. PMID: 25814028. PMCID: PMC4386321

[34] Nowosielski M, Galldiks N, Iglseder S, Kickingereder P, von Deimling A, Bendszus M, et al. Diagnostic challenges in meningioma. Neuro-Oncology. 2017;**19**(12):1588-1598

[35] Goldbrunner R, Minniti G, Preusser M, Jenkinson MD, Sallabanda K, Houdart E, et al. EANO guidelines for the diagnosis and treatment of meningiomas. The Lancet Oncology. 2016;**17**(9):e383-e391

[36] Lyndon D, Lansley JA, Evanson J, Krishnan AS. Dural masses: Meningiomas and their mimics. Insights into Imaging. 2019;**10**(1):11

[37] Lee EJ, Park JH, Park ES, Kim JH. "wait-and-see" strategies for newly diagnosed intracranial Meningiomas based on the risk of future observation failure. World Neurosurgery. 2017;**107**:604-611

[38] Zhao L, Zhao W, Hou Y, Wen C, Wang J, Wu P, et al. An overview of managements in Meningiomas. Frontiers in Oncology. 2020;**10**:1523

[39] Preusser M, Brastianos PK, Mawrin C. Advances in meningioma genetics: Novel therapeutic opportunities. Nature Reviews Neurology. 2018;**14**(2):106-115

Chapter 2

Diagnosis and Grading of Meningiomas

Frank Y. Shan, Dongxia Feng, Yilu Zhang, Karming Fung, Jennifer H. Murillo and Jason H. Huang

Abstract

Meningiomas are the most common primary brain tumors in adults. They are slow growing, mostly benign tumors affecting primarily older people. Meningiomas comprise a family of neoplasms that are most likely derived from the meningothelial cells of the arachnoid cap cell. Current diagnosis of meningioma has been facilitated by MRI scans, and most patients with meningiomas have good prognosis without affecting the quality of life after successful treatment, like gross total resection (GTR). This chapter will briefly review the molecular basis, clinical diagnosis and grading of meningiomas and the treatment options.

Keywords: meningioma, dura-based tumors, dural tail sign, DNA methylation, metastatic carcinoma

1. Introduction

Meningiomas are the most common primary brain tumors, which are primarily benign neoplasms affecting mainly elderly population with a median age of 66 years [1]. Meningioma occurs in the USA at an average annual age-adjusted rate of 8.58 cases per 100,000 population, accounting for 37.6% of CNS tumors. Although this tumor more commonly occurs in the elderly patients, it has a preference to affect the young population, especially women during pregnancy. This tumor is often described as an extra-axial tumor, but location of tumor still plays an important role in treatment and prognosis. As the improvement of diagnostic and treatment methods, this tumor should become a manageable neoplasm.

2. Incidence and etiology of meningiomas

Meningioma is the single most common tumor reported in patients older than 35 years. The incidence of meningioma is about 5.35 per 100,000 person years (3.17 in males and 7.19 in females), with a mean age at diagnosis of 64 years [1]. The incidence of meningioma is increasing, probably due to the incidental finding of this tumor by radiologic examination, as the technology becomes more advanced. Another

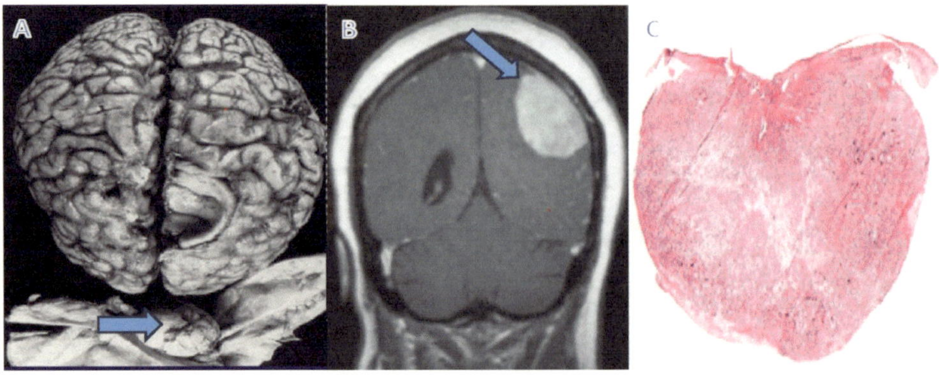

Figure 1.
Incidental finding of a meningioma during autopsy, arrow (A), tumor made a dent in brain tissue. (B) CT scan of a left frontal meningioma, the arrow indicates the dural tail. The tumor had mass effect to push the lateral ventricle. A gross picture of a resected meningioma attached to the dura (C).

incidental finding of meningioma is by autopsy, in which removing the brain may lead to finding of meningioma attached to the skull (**Figure 1A**).

Exposure to ionizing radiation is the primary and established risk factor for meningioma, especially those who were exposed in childhood. In addition, several findings suggested a risk association between hormone and meningioma, including the greater incidence of meningioma in women than in men, and the presence of hormonal receptors in some meningiomas, as well as a modestly increased risk associated with endogenous and exogenous hormone. Hormone-related risk of meningiomas was also found in patients treated with progestin, and patients with uterine fibroid, endometriosis, and breast cancer. Other attempts to link specific chemicals, diet, occupation, head trauma, and mobile phone use with meningioma have been inconclusive so far [1].

3. Clinical presentation of meningiomas

Clinical presentation of meningiomas varies based on the location of the tumor. Headache is a common symptom, and it may worsen with time. When tumor affects the brain surface (cortex), seizure may occur. In some elderly patients with cerebral atrophy, the symptoms may be mild, as there is more space for tumor growth until it reaches the surface of the brain. When the tumor compresses cranial nerves, especially in skull base meningiomas, nerve-damage-related symptoms may occur. As an example, the anterior fossa meningioma compresses the olfactory nerve leading to loss of smell, while compressing the optic nerve may lead to blurred, or double vision, or even blindness, and exophthalmos (**Figure 2A**). While tumors in the sella turcica region may cause visual field defect due to optic chiasm damage as well as abnormal hormonal expression by compressing the pituitary gland.

In the current WHO Classification of CNS tumors [1], meningiomas have 3 grades, primarily based on histopathological evaluation and their clinical behavior. These gradings are closely related to the clinical behavior of meningiomas including the recurrence rate. Grades 1, 2 and 3 meningiomas have 5-year recurrence rate of 12%, 41%, and 56% [2], respectively.

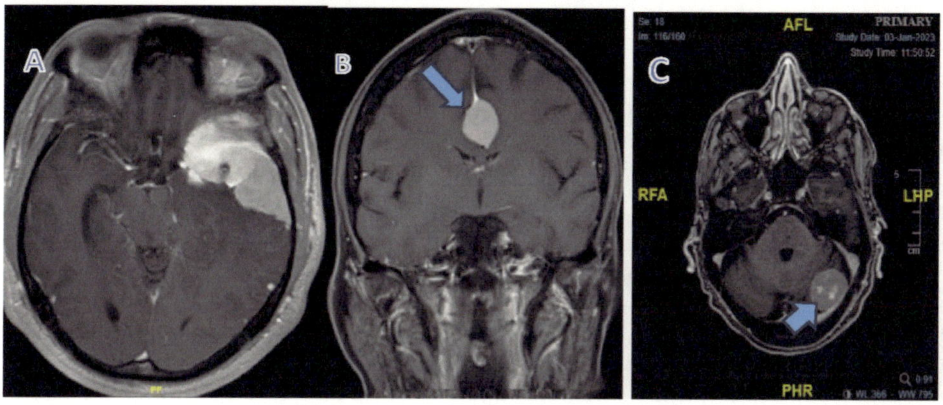

Figure 2.
Middle cerebral fossa tumor with an en plaque meningioma, with no dual tail (A); parafalcine meningioma is close to superior sagittal sinus, arrow (B); uncommon cerebellar meningioma with dural tail sign, arrow (C).

Meningiomas often have dural invasion, and to prevent tumor recurrence, resection of a segment of dura is necessary (**Figure 1C**).

4. Location of meningiomas

As with most diseases in central nerve system (CNS), location is an important factor in clinical presentation and treatment of brain tumors. In meningiomas, location is not only related to the treatment option, but also has some genetic background, and affects the prognosis. The most common locations of meningiomas include the cerebral convexities, in association with the falx cerebri and/or venous sinuses, olfactory grooves, sphenoid ridges, tentorium, and posterior fossa. Intraventricular and epidural locations are uncommon. Especially the intraventricular meningioma, the origin the tumor is still a mystery. Most spinal meningiomas occur in the thoracic spine. Of note, convexity meningiomas and most of the spinal meningiomas carry a *22q* deletion and/or *NF2* mutations. Whereas skull base meningiomas harbor mutations in *AKT1, TRAF7, SMO,* and /or *PIK3CA*. High grade meningiomas more commonly arise from the convexity and other non-skull base sites. Rare primary meningiomas arise outside the CNS, including the lung, or skin.

Although it is called dura-based tumor, as a matter of fact, there are two more layers of membrane between dura and brain, they are arachnoid and pie membrane, collectively called "leptomeninges".

5. Molecular genetics of meningiomas

Monosomy of chromosome 22 is the most common genetic abnormality found in meningiomas, with more than half of the tumors showing allelic losses in 22q12.2. This region encodes the *NF2* gene. Initiation and malignant progression of *NF2*-driven meningiomas has been confirmed by animal models. While those meningiomas without *NF2* mutation, mutations of *AKT1* and *p.E17K* have been found. Since those mutations have been discovered in other cancers, they are considered as an oncogenic deriver. Additional genetic changes occur in higher grade meningiomas, with losses of 1p, 6p/q, 10q, 14q, and 18p/q; as well as less frequently losses of 2p/q, 3p, 4p/q, 7p, and 8p/q. In addition, *CDKN2A* and *CDKN2B* heterozygous or homozygous deletion have been reported. Moreover, *PIK3CA* mutations are associated with antihormone treatment. Women with meningioma who were under long-term progestin therapy carry *PIK3CA* mutations more frequently than those without hormone therapy, and high-dose antiandrogen treatment with cyproterone leads to an enrichment of *PIK3CA*-mutated skull base meningiomas [1].

More recently, DNA methylation profiling has become one of the most promising molecular tests for CNS tumors, and DNA methylation will be a new classification of CNS tumors in the near future [3]. A European study found that DNA methylation-based meningioma classification captures more homogenous groups and has a higher power for predicting tumor recurrence and prognosis than the current WHO classification [3, 4].

CDKN2A and *CDKN2B* are tumor suppressor genes, and studies showed that *CDKN2A* homozygous deletion has occasionally been reported in atypical and anaplastic meningiomas and is considered as one of the genetic alterations commonly involved in their recurrence and malignant progression [5]. The homozygous deletion can be detected by the FISH method.

6. Neuroimaging

Neuroradiology is important in the diagnosis and planning the treatment of meningiomas and other brain tumors. Commonly, meningiomas are isodense to gray matter on noncontract computed tomography (CT), and T1-weighted magnetic resonance imaging (MRI), They are contrast enhancing on MRI, and even small tumors (~3 mm) can be detected on MRI after administration of contrast agent. The "dural tail" sign on neuroimage is a very useful feature in the diagnosis of meningioma, or to confirm that the mass lesion is truly an extra-axial (**Figure 2**) [6]. Although some rare dura-based masses may have the same feature, they are very rare.

There is a special type of meningioma called "Meningiomas en plaque (MEP)", which is a rare subtype of meningioma that comprises only 2–9% of all meningiomas. MEP are unique from the more common en masse meningiomas and are defined by their characteristic "carpet-like" invasion of adjacent bone, with extensive hyperostosis and dural thickening (**Figure 2A**).

7. Histopathological diagnosis and grading of meningiomas

7.1 Meningothelial whorl

A hallmark of meningiomas, composed of epithelial cells with conspicuous nuclear pseudo-inclusion, indistinct cellular borders aggregated into small sheet and large lobules, impart a syncytial feature, to concentric rings, which finally makes this characteristic histological feature, called "meningothelial whorl". The central part may become hyalinized and calcified into psammoma body (**Figure 3A**).

Diagnosis and grading of meningiomas mainly rely on histopathologic evaluation. Meningiomas have at least more than ten histologic subtypes, most are benign, but some of them are associated with aggressive clinical behavior which need to be upgraded (grade 2 or 3), although rare, identifying those histological types is important for additional treatment and predicting the prognosis. The current grading system is based on WHO Classification of Central Nervous System Tumours [1].

The grading of meningiomas dramatically changed in the late 90s. Since in a large-scale study, brain invasion (used to call it "malignant meningioma") had been found not that "malignant" behavior clinically, and was downgraded as grade 2 atypical meningioma. The current WHO grading of meningiomas has 3 grades, as CNS WHO grade 1, 2 and 3 [1, 2].

8. CNS WHO grade 1 meningiomas

The most common histopathological type of meningiomas is meningothelial type (characterized by meningothelial whorls) and transitional type (**Figure 3**) [3]. The tumor cells are often in a nodular pattern, compared to the sheet-like pattern in more aggressive tumors. Sometimes, those types can be found mixed. Other WHO grade 1 types of meningiomas include psammoma body type (mostly occurs in female patients and thoracic spine), microcystic, angiomatous, and secretory (**Figures 4** and 5). The diagnosis of grade 1 meningioma is based on presence of mitoses less than 4/10 High power view (HPV). Besides, bone and dural invasion are

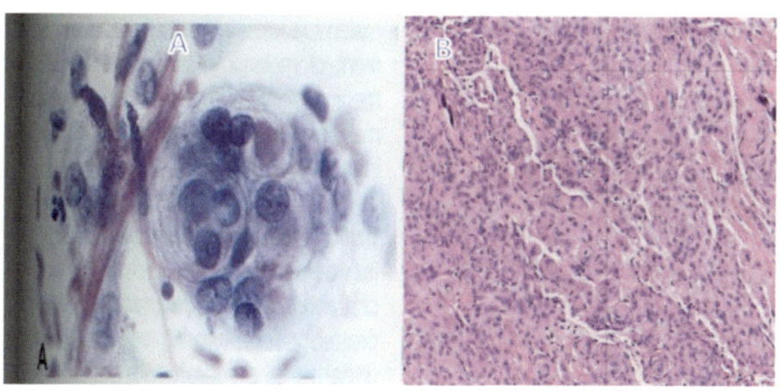

Figure 3.
Meningothelial whorl (A) is the diagnostic hallmark for meningioma H&E X400. Meningothelial meningioma with numerous meningothelial whorls (B, H&E X200).

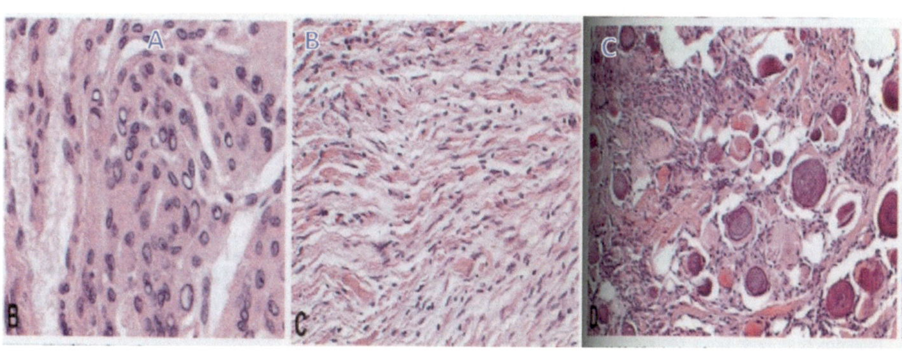

Figure 4.
Nuclear pseudo inclusion body is another histopathologic feature of meningioma (A). Fibrous meningioma with fibrous-like cells (B), psammoma body meningioma (C). All H&E X200.

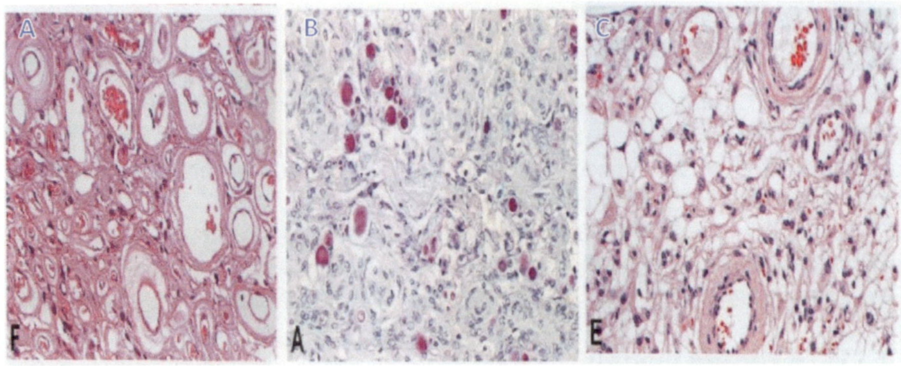

Figure 5.
Angiomatous (A), secretory (B) and microcystic (C) are other subtypes of grade 1 meningiomas. All H&E X200.

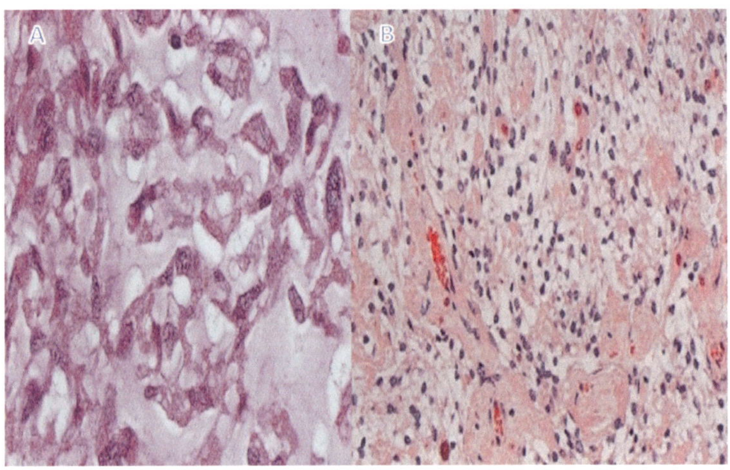

Figure 6.
Brain invasion is a diagnostic criterion for atypical meningioma. The tumor cells show penetrating rather than pushing feature into brain parenchyma (A H&E stain X200), confirmed by immunostaining of GFAP (brown color on the right indicating the brain parenchyma) (B, IHC stain X200).

still considered as grade 1 tumor. However, if the mitoses are more than 4 but less than 20 per 10 HPV, or the tumor has brain invasion, the tumor should be upgraded to WHO grade 2 atypical meningioma (**Figure 6**).

8.1 Meningothelial meningioma

The tumor is composed of numerous meningothelial whorls, as is categorized as grade 1 meningioma (**Figure 3**).

8.2 Fibrous meningioma

The tumor cells in this type of meningioma have spindle-cell features (**Figure 4B**), with collagen matrix surrounding the tumor cells. Some cases require immunohistochemical (IHC) stain to be distinguished from solitary fibrous tumor (SFT).

8.3 Transitional meningioma

Transitional meningioma is a mixture of both meningothelial and fibrous types, with focal whorls and psammoma bodies. This is the most common type of meningioma in practice.

8.4 Psammomatous meningioma

This subtype of meningioma mostly arises in the thoracic spine with female predominance and numerous Psammomatous calcification (**Figure 4C**).

8.5 Angiomatous meningioma

This subtype includes numerous capillary blood vessels with hyalinized vascular wall (**Figure 5A**). In some cases, nuclear atypia may be observed, which is not considered as a factor for higher grade, but a degenerative change.

8.6 Secretory meningioma

This subtype is characterized by round, eosinophilic periodic acid-Schiff (PAS)-positive, and carcinoembryonic antigen (CEA)-immunoreactive secretion (**Figure 5B**).

8.7 Microcystic meningioma

The microcystic change in this subtype is made by vacuolated tumor cells. Like with other brain tumors, microcystic feature is usually a sign of low-grade tumor, even in some cases, nuclear atypia and pleomorphism may be present, but it is not considered as a high grade feature (**Figure 5C**).

8.8 Metaplastic meningioma

This rare subtype may occasionally contain bone or cartilaginous, and lipomatous tissue, with no clinical significance.

8.9 Lymphoplasmacytic-rich meningioma

This rare subtype contains marked chronic inflammatory infiltrations, oftentimes obscuring the neoplastic meningioma cells, and makes the diagnosis challenging. However, in most meningiomas, some lymphocytes are always present.

8.10 CNS WHO grade 2 atypical meningiomas

Atypical meningiomas are associated with increased recurrence rate and seeding by cerebrospinal fluid (CSF), which need to be closely followed and adjuvant therapy might be necessary. The diagnoses of atypical meningiomas become more frequent, from 5–25% [6].

Specific histological subtypes related to atypical meningiomas inlude chordoid and clear cell types (**Figure 7**). In addition, brain invasion is one of the diagnostic criterion for atypical meningioma. Another diagnostic criterion for WHO grade 2

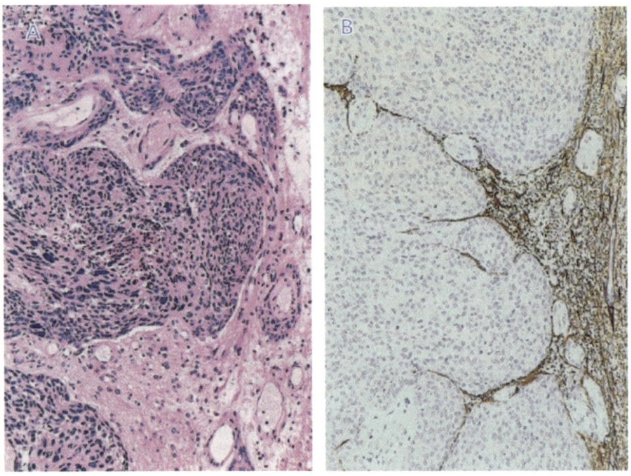

Figure 7.
Chordoid (A, H&E stain X400) and clear cell meningioma (B, H&E stain X200).

meningioma is increased mitoses more than 4/10 HPV but less than 20/10HPV. This needs careful microscopic evaluation [1]. Sometime, brain invasion needs immunohistochemical stain to be confirmed (**Figure 6**). Other less common histological criteria for atypical meningioma include focal necrosis, loss of nodular pattern with replacement of sheeting architecture, macronuclei, and small cell formation [6].

9. Histopathologic subtypes of WHO grade 2 meningiomas

9.1 Chordoid meningioma

This subtype of meningioma was named for its resemblance to the bone tumor, chordoma. Most cases are large, supratentorial masses and hard to resected. This tumor is composed of foamy or vacuolated "physaliferous-like" cells, often mixed with other types of meningiomas, making it hard to diagnose (**Figure 7A**).

9.2 Clear cell meningioma

This tumor is another subtype of grade 2 meningioma, it has a strong predilection to the spinal cord, and posterior fossa, as well as a younger age at presentation, and even happens in infants, children, and young adults [6]. The tumor is composed of sheets of cells with clear cytoplasm (**Figure 7B**), with almost no whorl and psammoma bodies. Immunohistochemical stains are usually required to separate it from metastatic clear cell renal cell carcinoma.

Brain invasion is another diagnostic criterion for CNS WHO grade 2 atypical meningioma. The brain invasion used to be called "malignant meningioma". It became less important after a large-scale study [2]. However, it carries some risk for recurrence, so it was categorized into grade 2 tumor. Careful evaluation of brain invasion is important in daily practice, and sometime immunohistochemical stains are required to differentiate true invasion from push artifact (**Figure 6**).

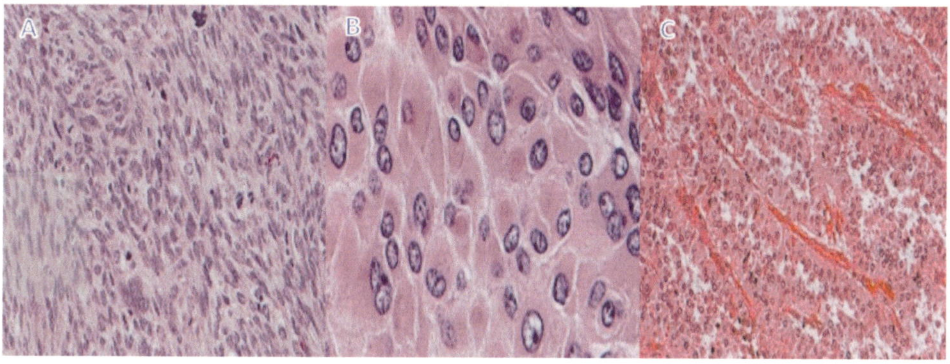

Figure 8.
Anaplastic (grade 3) meningioma with increased mitoses (A, H&E X200), Rhabdoid meningioma (B, H&E X400) and papillary meningioma (C, H&E X200).

10. CNS WHO grade 3 anaplastic meningioma

Grade 3 meningioma is essentially a malignant tumor, with increased recurrence rate and CSF seeding, as well as a poor prognosis. Although rare, identifying this type of tumor is very important. The specific histological subtypes related to anaplastic meningioma include rhabdoid and papillary (**Figure 8B** and **C**) meningiomas. In addition, mitoses more than 20/10HPV is considered as anaplastic feature (**Figure 8A**). Besides, their morphology can resemble carcinoma, sarcoma or even melanoma [3]. Molecular analysis plays an important role in assistance for diagnosis and predicting the prognosis of the anaplastic meningiomas, including telomerase reverse transcriptase (TERT) promoter mutation and homozygous deletion of *CDKN2A* and/or *CDKN2B* [3].

10.1 Rhabdoid meningioma

It is an aggressive meningioma with an ill-defined eosinophilic cytoplasmic inclusion, globular or fibrillar in texture. Often with necrosis and active mitotic activity (**Figure 8B**). In tumor pathology, almost all tumors with rhabdoid features have aggressive behavior and poor prognosis.

10.2 Papillary meningioma

This rare subtype of meningioma, like other papillary tumors, has a fibrovascular core, and the tumor cells have a perivascular arrangement of epithelial tumor cells resembling the pseudo rosettes of ependymoma (**Figure 8C**). This subtype of tumor has a potential to recurrence and metastasis to other organs [6]. Extracranial metastases to lung, pleura, bone and liver are rare but most often associated with CNS WHO grade 3 meningiomas. In one series, the incidence of metastases from all meningiomas was 0.67%, with a greater incidence in CNS WHO grade 2 and grade 3 meningiomas [1].

11. Other dura-based tumors like meningioma

Both solitary fibrous tumor (SFT) and hemangiopericytoma (HPC) used to be subtypes of meningiomas. They have been separated from meningioma due to different molecular genetics and immunohistochemical staining patterns. Those two tumors are positive for CD34 and with nuclear expression of STAT6 by immunohistochemical stain and both have fusion of *NAB2* and *STAT6*. Currently, these two tumors are considered as one entity with different presentation, while SFT is in the benign end, the HPC is more aggressive and has frequent recurrence [1]. In addition, they may occur in the other organs of the human body.

12. Metastatic carcinomas to meninge and meningioma

Both breast cancer and prostate cancer have great potential to metastasis to dura. The breast cancer, followed by lung adenocarcinoma are the tumors documented most likely to metastasizes into meningioma, probably due to the hormonal reason. Those so-called collision tumors may cause some diagnostic difficulty, and immunohistochemical stains are required to detect the primary tumor (**Figure 9B**).

12.1 Skull-base meningiomas

Skull-base meningioma has its growth and histopathologic characteristics with different treatment methods. It leads to functional disturbance which significantly alters the quality of life. Although no being set up as a subtype, it is worth mentioning here.

The skull base is the floor, or base, of the skull located behind the eyes and nose, composed of five bones – the frontal, ethmoid, sphenoid, temporal and occipital – that provide support to the bottom of the brain, and contains many bony structures, blood vessels and nerves. The skull base is also called "fossa" and are separated into 3 fosses, including anterior, middle and posterior fosses. The anterior and middle fosses usually referred as "supratentorial". While the posterior fossa (inferior tentoria) contains cerebellum, part of brainstem and 4th ventricle, meningiomas may happen in posterior fossa although relatively uncommon (**Figure 2C**). Middle cerebral fossa meningioma may cause hearing loss or ringing in the ears, memory loss or weakness of arms and legs. Due to the complex bony structure, vessels and nerves, complete resection (GTR) of skull-base meningiomas may sometimes be challenging.

Middle cerebral fossa tumors may cause memory loss, and hearing defect, while posterior fossa tumors can lead to hearing defect, and dizziness.

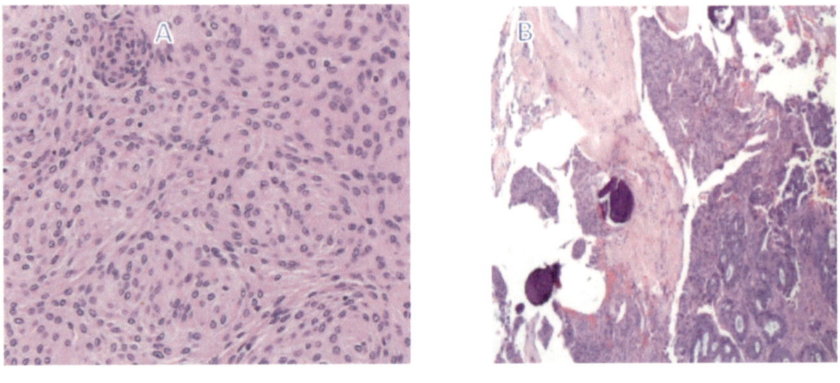

Figure 9.
Skull-base meningioma is with incomplete whorl as a nodule (A, H&E X200), a collision tumor of metastatic adenocarcinoma of lung primary into meningioma (B, H&E X200).

Skull base meningiomas may have different histopathologic features compared to the convexity meningiomas, such as, skull-base meningioma has less well-formed meningothelial whorls (**Figure 9A**), compared to complete meningothelial whorls as seen in (**Figure 3A** and **B**), probably due to its growth condition, but the incomplete larger nodules resemble the whorls (**Figure 9A**).

13. Clinical management of meningiomas

Management of meningiomas varies based on several factors, including the extent and severity of symptoms and signs, tumor size and location. Some meningiomas are asymptomatic while other tumors can cause location-specific neurologic deficits, general non-specific symptoms or both. Location-specific symptoms can result in visual disturbances, hearing loss, aphasia, hemiparesis or hemi-sensory changes. More generalized symptoms that frequently occur include headache, nausea/vomiting, dizziness, and seizures. Seizures occur in 30–40% of meningioma patients [7].

Meningioma management can include observation by monitoring the tumor with regular imaging. Some meningiomas are followed by observation, particularly those that are small, incidental, and asymptomatic in nature. For larger, symptomatic tumors or for tumor progression or in tumor recurrence, the two most common treatment modalities include surgery and radiation therapy. Chemotherapy is becoming a more common treatment modality in recurrent meningiomas with an increase in molecular testing for targeted treatment.

Surgical resection is the primary treatment modality in symptomatic tumors. Careful consideration is required to determine if symptoms can be localized to the tumor or associated peritumor edema. The tumor location, amount of safe resection and the patient's overall health, including medical comorbidities, age, and performance status are used to determine the surgical risk vs. benefit for tumor resection. The surgical approach varies based on tumor size and location. Meningiomas that are located along the convexity of the calvaria vault are more accessible but are also associated with an increased risk of vascular injury in midline convexity tumors due to the proximity to major venous sinuses like the superior sagittal sinus. Meningiomas that grow along the base of the skull also pose an increased risk of a neurologic deficit given the proximity and involvement of cranial nerves and vessels that transverse the skull at its base [8].

The second common treatment approach includes radiotherapy. Radiotherapy is typically considered as the primary treatment if the tumor is not able to be safely resected based on the location, size, or when a patient is a poor surgical candidate to obtain disease control. Additionally, radiation therapy is also considered post-surgically if maximal resection is not achieved, tumor has recurrence or in cases of inoperable locations, and high grades. Radiosurgery or stereotactic radiotherapy in single or multiple doses may be appropriate in small tumors whereas external beam radiotherapy is more appropriate for recurrent, multiple or extensive lesions with a dose of up to 70 Gy for grade 2/3 meningiomas [9].

The use of chemotherapy in meningiomas remains an area of unmet need. Chemotherapy is typically used in the treatment of recurrent meningioma supported by national comprehensive cancer network (NCCN) guidelines, with several options including sunitinib, bevacizumab, octreotide, and combination therapy like bevacizumab combined with everolimus. Additional research is needed to identify potential targeted treatment based on the molecular characteristics and the genetic mutations previously associated with meningiomas including *NF2, SMO, TERT,* and *TRAF7* [9].

Symptom management in meningiomas can be challenging. Several common neurological symptoms seen in this patient population include seizures, headaches and mood disorders. Brain tumor-related seizures can be treated with anti-epileptic medication or surgery to reduce tumor burden and to relieve associated mass effect. Anticonvulsant is typically recommended in patients with brain tumor who have experienced at least one seizure. There is no consensus on antiepileptic medication selection as several factors must be taken into consideration including age, psychological history and drug-drug interactions. New generation of anticonvulsants like levetiracetam, lacosamide, clobazam and vigabatrin are typically used as the first line with fewer drug-drug interactions [10]. Headaches are usually multifactorial but a high percentage of headaches in brain tumors are associated with vasogenic edema. As such, careful consideration of treatment options must be exercised when treating headaches. Corticosteroids effectively reduce cerebral edema and are often used in patients with brain tumor. Dexamethasone is often chosen for its long biological half-life, and low mineralocorticoid activity [11]. Mood disorders are also commonly seen in brain tumor patients. Mood disorder can be related to the direct tumor effect on neurologic functions, although the exact relationship between mood and tumor location remains unclear. Additionally, mood disorders can be triggered or exacerbated by medications, including steroids and antiepileptic medications like levetiracetam, making these disorders challenging to treat effectively. Typical medications used in the meningioma include antidepressants (SSRIs), antipsychotics, mood stabilizers or anxiolytic agents [11].

In conclusion, meningiomas are very common primary brain tumors. Its molecular genetics, clinical presentation, diagnosis and grading have been studied for a while, and the standard of care has been well-established. New information, especially molecular information becomes more and more commonly used in our practice, which provides new insight into this tumor. We believe as more information helps us to understand this tumor, it will become a manageable tumor soon.

Abbreviations

CNS	Central nervous system
CSF	Cerebrospinal fluid
SSS	Superior sagittal sinus
MRI	Magnetic resonance imaging
CT	Computed tomography
WHO	World Health Organization
FISH	Fluorescent in situ hybridization
GTR	Gross total resection
HPV	High power view
MEP	Meningioma en plaque
IHC	Immunohistochemical stain
GFAP	Glial fibrillary acidic protein
NF2	Neurofibromatosis 2

Author details

Frank Y. Shan[1,2*], Dongxia Feng[2], Yilu Zhang[2], Karming Fung[3], Jennifer H. Murillo[2] and Jason H. Huang[2]

1 Department of Anatomic Pathology, Baylor Scott and White Health, Baylor College of Medicine, Temple, TX, USA

2 Department of Neurosurgery, Baylor Scott and White Health, Baylor College of Medicine, Temple, TX, USA

3 Department of Pathology, University of Oklahoma Health Sciences Center, Oklahoma City, OK, USA

*Address all correspondence to: yshan918@gmail.com

References

[1] International Agency for Research on Cancer. WHO Classification of Tumours, Editorial Board, Central Nervous System Tumours. 5th ed. Lyon, France: International Agency for Research on Cancer; 2021

[2] Perry A, Stafford SL, Scheithauer BW, Suman VJ, Lohes CM. Meningioma grading: An analysis of histologic parameters. American Journal of Surgical Pathology. 1997;**21**(12):1455-1465

[3] Davidson C. Histopathologic and molecular evaluation of meningioma. Neurosurgery Clinics of North America. 2023;**34**:311-318

[4] Sahm F, Schrimpf D, et al. DNA-methylation-based classification and grading system for meningioma: A multicentre, retrospective analysis. The Lancet Oncology. 2017;**18**:682-694

[5] Shoh S, Maiko T, Takanori H, Tomomi F, Hiroe I, Tomoko U, et al. Correlation of MTAP immuno-histochemistry with CDKN2A status assessed by fluorescence In situ hybridization and Clinicopathological features in CNS WHO grade 2 and 3 Meningiomas: A single Center cohort study. Journal of Neuropathology and Experimental Neurology. 2022;**81**(2):117-126

[6] Perry A, Brat DJ. Expert Consult: Practical Surgical Neuropathology, a Diagnostic Approach. Churchill Livingstone; 2010

[7] Englot DJ, Chang EF, Vecht CJ. Epilepsy and brain tumors. Handbook of Clinical Neurology. 2016;**134**:267-285

[8] Bi WL, Dunn IF. Current and emerging principles in surgery for meningioma. Chinese Clinical Oncology. 2017;**6**(Suppl. 1):S7

[9] Apra C, Peyre M, Kalamarides M. Current treatment options for meningioma. Expert Review of Neurotherapeutics. 2018;**18**(3):241-249

[10] Lee EQ. Neurologic complications in patients with cancer. Continuum (Minneap Minn). 2020;**26**(6):1629-1645

[11] Forst DA. Palliative and supportive care in neuro-oncology. Continuum (Minneap Minn)

Chapter 3

Quality of Life in Patients with Meningioma

Mohsen Merati, Fateme Montazeri, Farnam Mohebi, Hannaneh Kabir and Hamidreza Komaki

Abstract

Meningiomas are common benign brain tumors that may significantly impact patients' Health-Related Quality of Life (HRQOL) and functional disability. The assessment of HRQOL in meningioma patients is heterogeneous, necessitating standardized approaches. Patient-Reported Outcome Measures (PROMs) are increasingly used to capture patients' perspectives, with various questionnaires developed for this purpose. Medical and non-medical risk factors for long-term HRQOL impairment encompass tumor characteristics, treatment factors, and sociodemographic features. Symptomatic meningioma patients experience lower HRQOL scores, with symptoms influenced by tumor features such as location, edema, and size. Prominent subsequent manifestations, including epilepsy, neurocognitive dysfunction, and psychiatric symptoms, significantly influence HRQOL. Surgical resection is the primary therapeutic option, and adjuvant radiotherapy may be considered for recurrent or high-risk cases. Although patients generally experience improved HRQOL post-surgery, some may face long-term declines, necessitating comprehensive long-term well-being evaluation. Patients often undergo positive changes in mental outlook (posttraumatic growth), triggering a "response shift" that may alter patients' values and internal standards, ultimately improving their perception of HRQOL. Long-term outcomes highlight meningioma's chronic impact on patients' lives and socioeconomic burden. Overall, understanding and addressing these factors optimizes patients' well-being and functional outcomes. A holistic approach considering medical and psychosocial aspects is crucial for enhancing HRQOL in meningioma patients.

Keywords: meningioma, health-related quality of life (HRQoL), patient-reported outcome measures (PROMs), socioeconomic burden, risk factors, long-term outcomes, inequality

1. Introduction

Meningiomas stand as one of the most common types of primary brain tumors, constituting about a third of all tumors within the central nervous system. Most meningiomas are histologically benign, asymptomatic, and frequently detected during medical evaluations for other conditions. Incidental asymptomatic meningiomas do not induce a mass effect and may thus have no impact on a patient's quality of

IntechOpen

life [1]. However, symptomatic patients experience a broad spectrum of neurological and psychological manifestations. These symptoms primarily arise from mass pressure exerted on surrounding tissues, induced seizures, or treatment complications [2]. Based on tumor location, symptoms include visual impairment, cognitive disturbance, psychiatric symptoms, and neuropathies. It is also common for patients to report non-specific symptoms like sleep disturbances, fatigue, and psychosocial challenges.

Advancements in radiation and surgical techniques have remarkably improved the prognosis for patients diagnosed with meningiomas. According to prior studies, meningioma patients' life expectancy approaches the general population, with 5-year survival rates at 92% (as opposed to the expected survival of 94%) and 10-year survival rates at 81% (versus the expected survival of 86%). However, patient functionality is inevitably impacted by the physical and cognitive symptoms associated with meningiomas, leading to inherent limitations in their daily lives, which substantially reduce their life quality [2]. For instance, a significant proportion, approximately two-thirds of patients, persistently suffer from moderate to severe neurological deficits even 5 years post-surgery [3]. However, the importance of these functional issues may be underestimated in the treatment strategies implemented by neurosurgeons, radiotherapists, or oncologists [4]. To many patients, the quality of life during and after treatment holds equal importance as treating their cancer and plays an important role in the patient's overall outcomes [5]. Therefore, a paradigm shift in current therapeutic goals for meningiomas is necessary, moving away from a singular focus on survival and surgical tumor resection toward a more holistic approach with prioritizing patients' performance and life satisfaction.

Recently, health-related quality of life (HRQoL) has been introduced as a meaningful indicator in cancer management. It is a comprehensive concept that encompasses various dimensions of life contributing to subjective physical, mental, and social well-being. Multiple measurement methodologies have been developed to gather clinical history and evaluate patients' HRQoL. However, certain aspects with considerable short and long-term impacts on daily life, such as cognitive impairment, memory loss, and personality changes, remain challenging to objectively quantify [4].

This chapter aims to delve into HRQoL in patients with meningiomas, shedding light on how the disease and its treatments can influence HRQoL. Our exploration will encompass various aspects of HRQoL in meningioma patients, ranging from HRQoL assessment, risk factors, impacts on cognitive and psychiatric functions, immediate and long-lasting outcomes of treatments, associated socioeconomic burden, HRQoL inequality, and also application of artificial intelligence in prediction of HRQoL.

2. Assessment of health-related quality of life

In recent years, there has been a growing inclination toward understanding the HRQoL and functional disability that meningioma patients have experienced [6]. Quality of life (QoL) is influenced by multiple factors within cultural frameworks that shape the patients' objectives and perspectives. Standard indicators of QoL should consider diverse elements, such as patient environment, level of education, and even leisure time activities, in addition to physical and mental health status [6]. Current reports of QoL among meningioma patients have employed heterogeneous methodologies, with different scales and follow-up protocols, which highlights the importance of developing standardized approaches to evaluate long-term functionality and QoL, particularly among those who have been surgically treated [1].

A significant challenge in this regard is the lack of available data regarding the long-term functional outcomes of patients with meningiomas. Conventional outcome measures such as complications, extent of resection, and survival rates can be ascertained by healthcare providers. However, the data concerning quality of life should ideally be reported by the patients themselves [6]. Patient-reported outcomes are gaining importance and are rapidly becoming the most precise and reliable reflections of the patient's perspectives [7]. Several self-assessment questionnaires have been developed specifically for patients to report their experiences and perceptions of HRQoL. These questionnaires, commonly recognized as patient-reported outcome measures (PROMs), constitute a valuable instrument for capturing the subjective history and perspectives of patients, ensuring that their experiences are not only acknowledged but also duly considered in the comprehensive evaluation of their HRQoL [1, 6].

Table 1 illustrates some examples of HRQoL assessment tools. Among them, the National Institute of Health Patient-Reported Outcomes Measurement Information System (PROMIS) provides instruments that can be customized according to specific requirements. Another assessment tool is the Short Form 36 (SF-36) questionnaire,

Instrument Specificity	Name of Questionnaires	Assessment of Medical Conditions	What is measure?	Subdomains
Generic	SF-36	Evaluating the health status of individuals, commonly used in health economic analysis for cost-effectiveness assessment	A set of 36 items centered on patient-reported physical functioning and role limitations	Role limitations, pain, overall health perception, physical functioning, vitality, social interaction, overall mental well-being
	PROMIS	Highly pertinent and applicable to both chronic and acute medical conditions	Assessment of patient-reported physical, mental, and social capabilities	Fatigue, pain severity, pain disruption, physical functioning, sleep disruption, anxiousness, despondency, and role restrictions
	EQ-5D	Applied in population health investigations, clinical trials, and economic assessments with wide-ranging relevance	A detailed descriptive examination of five subcategories paired with an appraisal of general health status through the use of the visual analog scale (VAS)	Mobility, self-care, typical activities, pain/discomfort, anxiety/depression (mental distress)
Brain Tumor	FACT-BR	Individuals receiving therapy for glioma	44 items, patient reported	Physical, emotional, and functional health, along with any additional symptoms

Instrument Specificity	Name of Questionnaires	Assessment of Medical Conditions	What is measure?	Subdomains
	MDASI-BT	Individuals receiving treatment for glioma	22 items, patient reported	General, localized, and treatment-associated symptoms encountered in the preceding 24 hours
	BN20	Individuals receiving treatment for glioma	10 items, patient reported	Future uncertainty, visual impairments, motor dysfunction, speech challenges, emotional distress, and symptoms specific to brain tumors
	EORTC QLQ-BN20	Individuals receiving treatment for glioma	20-Item supplement to EORTC QLQ-C30	Future uncertainty, visual impairment, motor impairment, communication difficulties, headaches, seizures, drowsiness, hair loss, itching, leg weakness, and bladder control issues
Cancer	EORTC QLQ-C30	A range of cancer types, encompassing lung, breast, gynecologic, prostate, colorectal cancer, and brain tumors	30 cancer-related items, patient reported	Physical, role, cognitive, emotional, and social functioning, along with fatigue, nausea, vomiting, and pain
Functional Disability	KPS	Created for medical practitioners to gauge a patient's cancer survival potential, utilizing a scale where 0 indicates mortality and 100 signifies a state of well-being with no complaints and no signs of disease		

Abbreviations: EQ-5D, EuroQol 5 Dimension; MDASI-BT, M.D. Anderson Symptom Inventory-Brain Tumor; EORTC QLQC30, European Organization for Research and Treatment of Cancer Quality of Life Questionnaire Version 3; KFS, Karnofsky Performance Status; EORTC QLQ-BN20, Quality of Life Questionnaire Brain Neoplasm Module 2.0; FACT-BR, Functional Assessment of Cancer Therapy Brain Module; PROMIS, National Institute of Health Patient-Reported Outcomes Measurement Information System; SF-36, Short Form Health Survey-36 item [1, 6, 8, 9].

Table 1.
Health-related quality of life and functional disability assessment tools.

which encompasses 36 self-reported items and has been widely utilized as the primary method for assessing QoL. Beyond just measuring health status, SF-36 facilitates health economics analysis and supports the calculation of cost-effectiveness [1]. Another valuable tool is the Karnofsky Performance Scale (KPS) which is commonly used questionnaire for the assessment of functional decline in patients with advanced illnesses [6]. While these generalized assessment tools are designed to evaluate physical, cognitive, emotional, and social functioning across diverse populations, they do not specifically target central nervous system pathologies. This oversight creates a gap where specific concerns related to meningiomas remain unaddressed [10].

3. Risk factors (predictors) of long-term impairment of HRQoL

Besides the HRQoL assessment tools, specific factors come into play that aid in estimating and predicting the eventual severity of HRQoL impairment. Within clinical contexts, the identification of these risk factors serves as a crucial tool for effectively allocating treatment, rehabilitation, and supportive care services. This targeted approach ensures that those in most need receive the maximum benefits, thereby reducing the overall burden imposed by the disease [11].

3.1 Clinical risk factors

The long-term burden of meningioma has been determined by clinical risk factors including treatment characteristics and complications like surgery-related complications, reoperation, and radiotherapy, as well as tumor characteristics [11, 12]. An earlier study revealed negative associations between tumor diameter, tumor activities (as denoted by the presence of edema and a larger tumor diameter on the last MRI), and patients' executive functioning. Remarkably, the study demonstrated that 67% of meningioma patients suffered from neurocognitive deficits, which negatively impacted their HRQoL [11, 13].

In light of these findings, healthcare providers should place particular emphasis on these clinical risk factors when gathering patient history. This approach can provide valuable insights into the potential need for ongoing supportive care and rehabilitation interventions, which are vital components in enhancing the overall well-being of meningioma patients [11, 13].

3.2 Non-clinical risk factors

Moving beyond the clinical predictors, non-clinical ones in brain tumor surgeries have been relatively under-explored in research. However, understanding and considering these elements are essential for a comprehensive evaluation of patients undergoing neurosurgical interventions. These non-clinical predictors extend beyond medical and surgical considerations, integrating individual characteristics such as social, psychological, and cognitive elements. These factors are typically assessed by clinicians, while they can also be directly reported by patients through PROMs [14].

Predominant non-clinical predictors often encompass sociodemographic variables, including age, gender, household income, socioeconomic status, insurance coverage, and marital status. Psychological attributes, including the presence of depressive and anxiety symptoms, altered mental states, independence in daily activities, and personality typologies, have also emerged as notable non-medical predictors influencing HRQoL. Furthermore, cognitive functions encompassing language deficits, attention spans, executive functions, psychomotor velocity, global cognitive functioning, and working memory have been studied as salient predictors of postoperative outcomes [14].

Additionally, an extended follow-up period as a risk factor was also observed to have a positive correlation with enhanced long-term HRQoL, as quantified by the SF-36 questionnaire. Specifically, patients with meningiomas who scored beneath the 25th percentile of normative data on more than four subscales had an average follow-up duration of 2.9 years. Conversely, those scoring beneath the 25th percentile on fewer than four subscales reported an average follow-up duration of 5.4 years (p-value <0.05). Moreover, a prolonged postoperative period correlated with reduced emotional impairment among these patients [15, 16].

It is interesting to note that in the long-time monitoring of patients with meningioma, HRQoL outcomes of different studies have yielded conflicting findings with different risk factors. This may be influenced by psychological mechanisms related to coping with surgery and illness. Patients might undergo a positive mental transformation, known as posttraumatic growth, which is commonly observed in long-term follow-up of patients with various types of cancer or acquired brain injury. This growth in mental well-being may also lead to a "response shift," causing patients to experience changes in their values, internal standards, and, subsequently, their perception of HRQoL, ultimately contributing to an enhanced quality of life [17, 18].

4. Quality of life in symptomatic/asymptomatic patients

Some meningiomas remain asymptomatic or undetected during follow-up, while patients with symptomatic tumors often report lower health status compared to healthy individuals. These impairments, though subtle, can easily escape notice. In a specific study monitoring individuals with suspected meningiomas, a decrease in vitality and overall well-being was discerned. However, when examined through the SF-36 questionnaire, no statistically significant differences were found in physical function, physical discomfort, role limitations, emotional distress, social interactions, and mental health. The authors attribute these changes to the only awareness of having an intracranial tumor and its potential psychological impact on patients, resulting in lower scores for vitality and general health domains in the HRQoL assessment. Importantly, these changes could not be detected and explained by differences in neurocognitive test performance when compared to healthy controls [19]. These findings indicate that patients with meningiomas may not experience significant physical impairments directly linked to their tumors (asymptomatic); however, they may still suffer from psychological distress like depression and anxiety. Conversely, meningioma patients displaying clinical symptoms reported diminished scores in multiple domains when compared to healthy controls of the same age. These areas included self-care, cognition, vitality, physical health, working memory, verbal memory, psychomotor speed, and role limitations [20].

Symptomatic meningiomas suffer from a wide range of clinical severity and symptoms, largely dependent on their specific location within the brain. The most frequently observed anatomical sites for meningiomas are as follows: convexity (35%), parasagittal (20%), sphenoid ridge (20%), infratentorial (13%), and other locations (12%). These regions delineate clinically significant subgroups with unique pathological attributes and linked physical symptoms. For instance, a relatively small meningioma situated in the tuberculum area can affect vision. In contrast, a meningioma of similar size located in the infratentorial region can result in myelopathy at the craniocervical junction or lead to hearing loss when positioned in the cerebellopontine angle.

Another example is that meningiomas which are located at the skull base pose a higher inherent risk of surgical morbidity. This is primarily due to the narrow approaching corridors in that area, the close proximity to critical neurovascular structures, and the relatively delicate nature of lower cranial nerves when it comes to tolerating surgical intervention [21].

Furthermore, in meningioma patients, prevalent preoperative symptoms include alterations in vision, cranial nerve impairments, ambulation challenges, cognitive deterioration, and tinnitus. Among these, visual symptoms had the most pronounced impact on reducing HRQoL. It is worth noting that HRQoL scores were positively associated with optic nerve decompression and the absence of proptosis (eye bulging) [22].

It is strikingly important to understand that the broad range of symptoms is based on precise intracranial locations of the meningioma. This emphasizes the clinical significance of considering the distinct anatomical features and related physical manifestations in the diagnosis and treatment of patients with symptomatic meningiomas.

4.1 Neurocognitive functioning

Unfortunately, there is limited knowledge regarding the impact of neurocognitive dysfunction on HRQoL of patients with meningioma before their surgery. However, several studies exclusively have been done on supratentorial meningiomas, and consistently identified deficits in various domains of cognitive function, including fluency, working memory, attention, processing speed, extended reaction times, and elevated error rates, when comparing patients to healthy individuals [19, 23].

While neurocognitive impairments can endure in meningioma patients post-treatment, the majority of patients tend to see an enhancement in their HRQoL after surgery. In a study involving meningioma patients who underwent a comprehensive set of neuropsychological evaluations right after their surgeries, lower scores were evident in all cognitive domains, including cognitive flexibility, memory, reaction time, psychomotor speed, executive functioning, processing speed, and complex attention. However, when re-assessed using identical tests 3 months later, enhancements were observed in all cognitive areas except for psychomotor speed and reaction time [24].

4.2 Psychiatric manifestations

When it comes to psychiatric presentation, first, it is important to note that the degree of change in one's happiness (level of anxiety, depression, and happiness) around a "set point" would be influenced by the individual's capacity to adjust to their new medical condition. Elevated scores in emotional stability and awareness represent psychological factors linked to improved HRQoL, whereas cognitive dysfunction and diminished functionality contribute to a decline in HRQoL [25].

Some patients with primary brain lesions may show no clinical symptoms; however, others might have various presentations like seizures, headaches, alterations in baseline cognitive function, focal neurological deficits, and psychiatric manifestations. For individuals with a mental illness history, it becomes particularly challenging to differentiate between symptoms of a primary psychiatric condition and those caused by meningioma. For example, if a patient presents with the chief complaint of apathy, this symptom might be attributed only to major depressive disorder. In such a case where patients have a history of major depressive disorder and their presentation resembles previous episodes, additional diagnostic laboratory testing may not be requested. This is because patients with major depressive disorder are at a higher risk of recurrent depression, particularly if antidepressant medications have been discontinued for a while [26].

In terms of psychiatric symptoms, brain lesions can affect nearby neurons by compressing surrounding structures and then disrupting neuronal activity, which results in some psychiatric manifestations. There is a correlation between the location of brain tumors and the specific psychiatric symptoms they manifest [27]. For instance, frontal and temporal tumors tend to cause more psychiatric symptoms compared to those localized in the parietal and occipital lobes [26]. Also, previous literature reviews have consistently shown a correlation between frontal meningiomas and depressive symptoms and also highlighted a positive association between right frontal meningiomas and the prevalence of major depressive disorder, atypical depression, and psychosis [28–30].

All these findings emphasize the importance of considering tumor location when assessing psychiatric symptoms in patients with brain lesions, as it can provide valuable insights into potential associations between specific tumor sites and distinct psychiatric manifestations. Comprehensive evaluation and localization of brain lesions can help guide appropriate treatment strategies and enhance patient outcomes [31]. In this regard, the incorporation of neuroimaging into the assessment process of patients with atypical psychiatric symptoms, will help healthcare professionals to detect potential underlying brain lesions on time, and ultimately may lead to accurate and timely diagnosis [31].

4.3 Epilepsy

Seizures often present as an initial symptom in around 25–30% of individuals diagnosed with meningiomas [32, 33]. Several theories have been proposed to clarify the pathogenesis of brain tumor-related epilepsy in meningioma; however, there are still unresolved questions regarding the effective control and management of seizures in meningioma patients.

In terms of surgical management, on one hand, resection is often effective in reducing the use of antiepileptic drugs (AEDs), improving seizure control, and providing seizure freedom in a significant percentage of cases, ranging from 60–90% [34]. On the other hand, for about 12–19% of patients, seizures may persist even after the surgical procedure [35]. This is mostly due to the extent of tumor removal, which can predict the occurrence of postoperative seizures. These postoperative seizures can have adverse effects on a patient's quality of life, impacting their independence, cognitive functions, and ability to drive safely. In addition to the extent of tumor removal, there are other factors that may contribute to the risk of postoperative seizures. These factors encompass a prior history of preoperative language impairments, preoperative seizures, postoperative hydrocephalus, the use of postoperative anti-seizure medications, and the tumor's placement in the parietal region of the brain [36]. Also, there is a consistent association between seizures in meningioma and peritumoral edema and tumor location. In fact, peritumoral edema has been extensively studied and identified as the most robust predictor of seizures both before and after surgery [37].

Another research effort concentrated on supratentorial meningiomas in patients who experienced preoperative seizures. These patients were continually monitored, and it was found that around 90% of them attained freedom from seizures within 1 year following the surgical procedure. Factors associated with less favorable seizure control included a higher World Health Organization (WHO) grade, the presence of peritumoral edema exceeding 1 cm, incomplete tumor resection (Simpson III-IV), and tumor advancement during postoperative monitoring. Interestingly, findings revealed that patients with significant preoperative edema are less likely to achieve seizure freedom after surgery [36].

In terms of medical management, the reported efficacy of each individual antiepileptic drug (AED) varies widely in different studies. Among the medications studied in tumor-related epilepsy, levetiracetam and valproic acid have received the most extensive research and analysis [36], and it was observed that their usage can bring up detrimental effects on cognitive functions in some patients. In fact, epilepsy that begins at an earlier age and use of AEDs have both been associated with cognitive impairment and a lower quality of life. Irrespective of the underlying trigger for seizures, utilizing antiepileptic drugs (AEDs) and employing multiple medications (polypharmacotherapy) concurrently are robust indicators that negatively influence cognitive functioning in domains like processing speed, verbal understanding, and visuospatial capabilities [38].

Addressing polypharmacy issues related to AEDs is a complex and challenging decision that necessitates close collaboration between clinicians and patients. Several factors come into play, including the severity of the disease, medication side effects, and the patient's willingness to tolerate the risk of a potential breakthrough seizure. It is worth noting that the rate of post-withdrawal seizures remained consistent among patients who discontinued AEDs.

Several factors favor the continuation of AEDs, including the presence of preoperative seizures, the location of the tumor within the temporal region, a history of recurrent disease, and subtotal tumor resection. Overall, enhancing our comprehension and predictive capabilities regarding seizures in meningioma patients can guide health professionals to take effective seizure control approaches to improve HRQoL. Also, it enables a more accurate identification of patients at risk both before and after surgery [38].

5. Quality of life after treatments

The treatment of meningioma typically aims to preserve or enhance HRQoL. The extent of HRQoL improvement tends to vary based on the severity of symptoms prior to treatment [32]. Moreover, it is crucial to emphasize that several elements connected to meningiomas have shown a strong association with increased symptom distress even following treatment. These factors encompass tumor volumes exceeding 25 cc, frontal location, recurrent occurrences, incomplete resections, and lesions at the skull base, where achieving full tumor removal is frequently challenging [39].

Furthermore, the significance of PROMs has increased in various aspects of healthcare and medical research, particularly in assessing postoperative changes in the quality of life. Predicting the clinical course after surgery/radiotherapy remains challenging, but it holds paramount importance since patients often have unaddressed questions about their postoperative health status before undergoing surgery/radiotherapy. Besides this, understanding the factors associated with functional impairment after surgery/radiotherapy enables clinicians to enhance communication with patients during the preoperative evaluation process, leading to more informed decision-making, personalized interventions, and ultimately better patient care.

5.1 Surgery

Meningioma patients usually go through a positive clinical progression, where the treatment intensity is moderate and mainly involves neurosurgery. After mass resection, the majority of patients see an improvement in HRQoL and a reduction in pain, discomfort, and anxiety. However, some patients may experience a long-term decline in HRQoL, particularly in areas related to social and emotional functioning. To be more specific, various factors contributing to postoperative quality of life are as follows: burden of symptoms, age, size of tumor, histological grade, and extent of resection in surgery [39].

In one cross-sectional survey study, researchers have attempted to investigate socioeconomic burden and its impacts on quality of life in patients suffered from meningioma. They demonstrated remarkable improvements in specific scales of clinical symptoms after surgery. In **Figure 1a**, alterations in quality of life are illustrated

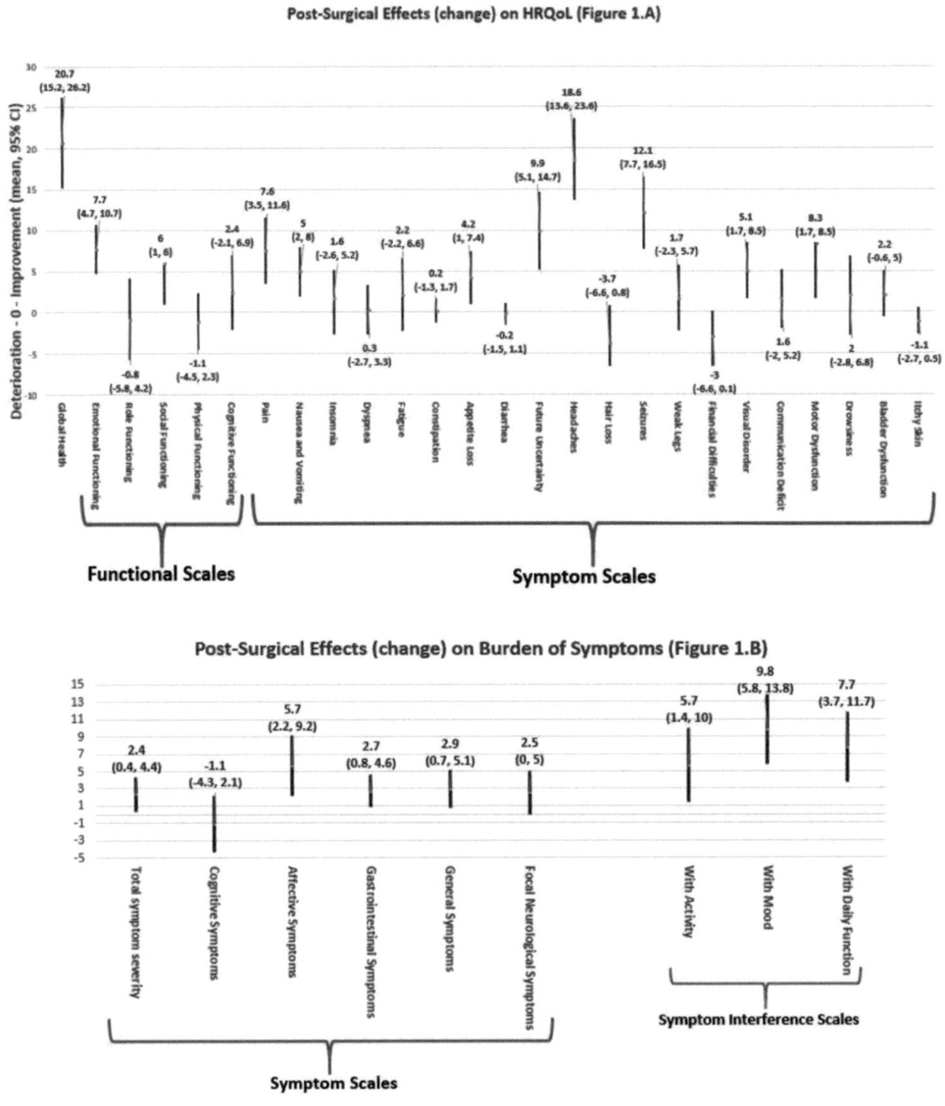

Figure 1.
Alterations in quality of life (A) and burden of symptoms (B) 1 year after meningioma surgery compared to pre-surgery condition [40]. Effect sizes were depicted through plots, which portray the variations in mean values on quasi-continuous scales spanning from 0 to 100. These effect sizes serve to visually convey the extent of changes in different aspects of patients' well-being and symptom experiences following surgery.

before and 1 year after surgery for patients with intracranial meningioma. These improvements are as follows: seizures (12.1%, 95% confidence interval (CI): 7.7–16.5%), headaches (18.6%, 95% CI: 13.6–23.6%), and global health (20.7%, 95% CI: 15.2–26.2%). However, there were less significant improvements (less than 10%) in future uncertainty, emotional and social functioning, and other different symptoms such as visual disorder, nausea and vomiting, pain, and appetite loss. Regarding the symptom burden, **Figure 1b** did not reveal any alterations exceeding 10% in symptom burden or interference. Nevertheless, it was observed that there were enhancements evident at lower levels across all scales except for cognitive functioning [40].

This research revealed a notable reduction in the workforce participation of patients, showing that 47 fewer individuals (20%) were currently employed. Among this group, 23 patients (10%) had retired as a result of age-related reasons ($p < 0.001$), 11 patients (5%) were dealing with disabilities, and 13 patients (5%) were without employment [40]. Among the initial 101 patients who were in full-time employment prior to their surgery, 21 individuals (21%) shifted to part-time employment, while 24 patients (24%) opted to cease working altogether. Among the 88 patients who were already working part-time before the procedure, 23 individuals (26%) also discontinued working. Consequently, there was an overarching decline in the number of patients engaged in full-time employment, while the number of those working part-time remained constant. Additionally, there was a rise of 21 patients (10%) who necessitated professional care ($p < 0.001$) [40]. The results of a binary regression analysis conducted on this cohort indicated that both occupational status (odds ratio [OR] of 0.41, 95% CI of 0.17–0.98, $p = 0.045$) and subjective ability to work (OR of 0.37, 95% CI of 0.15–0.92) were linked to a clinically significant decline in HRQoL. In fact, substantial proportion of meningioma patients (ranging from 19–35%) are unable to return to their pre-treatment level of employment [34].

In a study conducted by Miao, the HRQoL assessment tool with a 25-item questionnaire was used for both pre- and postoperative meningioma patients, as well as age-matched healthy individuals. The findings revealed that while HRQoL scores increased in meningioma patients following treatment, they still remained lower compared to the baseline HRQoL scores of the healthy controls [41]. Furthermore, analysis of clinical factors identified several significant predictors of HRQoL scores in meningioma patients. These predictors included tumor size (RR = 1.13), tumor recurrence (RR = 1.33), histologic grade (RR = 3.83), and tumor location (RR = 1.09). These findings provide strong evidence for the clinical factors that can impact HRQoL outcomes in surgeries [41].

Moreover, five predictors of functional impairment following brain tumor surgery have been identified in another research. These predictors include cranial nerve manipulation, major brain vessel manipulation, tumor size, posterior fossa location, and involvement of eloquent brain areas [42]. All these predictors could be combined and considered to monitor individuals in postsurgical periods, which enhances HRQoL and leads to better patient care.

5.2 Radiotherapy

However, surgical resection is often successful in curing the majority of cases. In a subgroup of patients with clinically aggressive meningioma, tumor recurrence may occur. Currently, no effective chemotherapy treatments are available for meningiomas. Instead, radiotherapy can be used to help control tumor growth in such cases. Generally, adjuvant radiotherapy is not typically administered after the complete removal of grade 1 meningiomas. Nonetheless, it is commonly integrated into the surgical strategy for grade II and III tumors or when dealing with recurring conditions [43].

A specific subgroup of meningioma patients, consisting of those with unresectable lesions or those with high risk for surgery, are suitable candidates for radiotherapy. Radiotherapy carries a relatively lower risk compared to surgery and demonstrates high rates of local tumor control. However, it is important to note that treatment-related toxicity can occur, including short-term neurological deficits associated with reactive edema and a few delayed neurocognitive effects [44].

Some previous research has focused on comparing the impact of adjuvant radiotherapy versus primary surgery without radiotherapy on HRQoL. The study results indicated that patients who underwent surgery followed by radiation treatment exhibited diminished HRQoL scores, especially in areas connected to memory, physical abilities, processing speed, and psychomotor speed. Nonetheless, when the groups were aligned based on demographic characteristics and the duration of the disease, these HRQoL score discrepancies vanished. This implies that the inclusion of radiotherapy following surgery does not result in extended adverse impacts on HRQoL [45, 46].

Despite potential short-term setbacks in verbal memory, working memory, and executive function, there have been observations of sustained or even enhanced HRQoL in the long run after skull-base meningioma removal and radiotherapy. This emphasizes the significance of conducting future studies to further investigate the long-term effects on HRQoL associated with different treatment options in patients with meningioma.

5.3 Short and long-term outcomes

Meningioma patients consistently exhibit lower scores of HRQoL compared to healthy individuals, both in the short and long term. Meningioma features such as edema, tumor size, and invasion impact patients in a manner similar to intramedullary brain tumors in a short time. In contrast, patients with minimal brain compression or those with tumors located near areas of the brain are more likely to experience minimal symptoms or remain asymptomatic [47].

In the long run, patients may consistently report ongoing reduction in HRQoL, particularly in the areas of social, emotional, cognitive, and executive functioning, even more than 120 months after their surgical treatment. It is important to note that the majority of HRQoL research focuses on grade 1 and 2 meningiomas. In this patient group, survival rates commonly exceed 10 years. Due to this prolonged survival, meningioma should be regarded as a chronic disease with persistent symptoms, emphasizing its long-term impact on patients' well-being and HRQoL [47].

6. Application of artificial intelligence in meningioma; using machine learning to predict HRQoL outcomes

Predicting HRQoL outcomes after the surgical removal of benign brain tumors serves a dual purpose: enabling early interventions and optimizing supportive care resource allocation. This proactive approach not only enhances clinical interventions but also empowers patients through education. Machine learning (ML), a subset of artificial intelligence (AI), equips systems with the capability to predict complex biological patterns that lack predefined models. Based on routine demographic and perioperative data, ML algorithms hold promise in predicting quality of life for patients with mild or benign brain tumors. These models offer potential to identify individuals prone to low levels of quality of life, facilitating efficient allocation of resource-intensive care [48].

While ML models have been applied to predict quality of life in cancer patients, none have been tailored for brain tumors [49]. Hence, the potential of ML in predicting HRQoL outcomes for low-grade meningiomas remains largely untapped. A recent breakthrough by Karri et al. utilizes an extensive dataset to explore various ML approaches, developing and assessing ten binary classifiers for quality-of-life prediction. These classifiers anticipate symptom presence or absence, as well as significant declines in overall quality of life relative to the population mean. The study covers a timeframe of 12 to 60 months after the removal of tumors. It makes use of data obtained from a longitudinal investigation conducted on patients who underwent surgery for low-grade glioma, meningioma, and acoustic neuroma at the Neuro-Oncology and Neurosurgery clinics of Royal Melbourne Clinic [50]. Derived from the QLQ-C30 questionnaire, a "global HRQoL" score forms the basis for a binary target variable. This variable identifies whether the global HRQoL score has dropped by at least 1 Minimal Clinically Important Difference (MCID) below the population mean of 75. Those meeting this threshold are labeled "1," signifying an expected lower HRQoL compared to the average population over time, while those above it are labeled "0." Using a chosen MCID of 10 points, aligned with previous studies, a "threshold" score of 65 is established [50].

Among six machine learning algorithms tested (Logistic Regression (LR), Decision Tree Classifier (DT), K Nearest Neighbors Classifier (KNN), Random Forest Classifier (RF), Support Vector Machine (SVM), and Gradient Boosting Machine (GBM)), the Support Vector Machine (SVM) emerges as the top performer for most outcomes. However, pain and diarrhea favor the Random Forest (RF) algorithm. This indicates the influence of hyperplane-based differentiation on predictive effectiveness across target variables. RF excels particularly for pain and diarrhea, indicating suitability for decision-tree-based differentiation [50]. In a broader context, predictive capacities of best-performing algorithms, measured by AUC (area under the curve), fall into three categories: >0.9, 0.8–0.9, or < 0.8. Metrics like appetite loss, constipation, nausea and vomiting, diarrhea, dyspnea, and fatigue exceed 0.9 AUC. Global HRQoL and financial difficulty score 0.8 to 0.9. In contrast, pain and insomnia consistently exhibit AUC below 0.8. PR-AUC (precision-recall area under the curve) scores echo AUC trends, deviating only for pain and diarrhea due to higher standard deviation during cross-validation [50].

Despite the potential shown by ML algorithms relying on routine demographic and perioperative data to forecast HRQoL outcomes for low-grade and benign brain tumors, limitations arise from derivation through a small-sample, single-center dataset. To enhance generalizability and account for symptom diversity across tumor types, expanded data collection on a multi-center scale is crucial. Such an approach would bolster algorithm applicability and refine predictions based on tumor-specific data.

7. Inequality in HRQoL of patients with meningioma

The complexities surrounding healthcare quality and equity are important issues. In recent years, there has been a growing focus and attention on disparities related to race, ethnicity, and socioeconomic factors within medical care. In this regard, limited research has addressed the influence of economic, social, cultural, and health system accessibility on the presentation of diseases and treatment outcomes, particularly concerning non-malignant tumors like intracranial meningioma. The assessment of healthcare equity holds the potential to mitigate discrepancies and enhance the standard of care for all individuals affected by intracranial meningioma.

The presence of inequalities in both disease presentation and treatment outcomes significantly impacts the well-being and survival of patients. In this context, studies have examined healthcare, demographic, and socioeconomic factors that contribute to diverse patient outcomes and HRQoL [51].

7.1 Socioeconomic factors

7.1.1 Impacts of socioeconomic factors on HRQoL

Various socioeconomic factors, such as income levels, educational attainment, and insurance coverage, have differing impacts on HRQoL, leading to disparities in HRQoL outcomes. In this context, a study conducted by Nayeri and colleagues in the United States, highlighted the influence of socioeconomic status on patient outcomes. Specifically, individuals with lower socioeconomic status, characterized by factors like Medicaid coverage and absence of a college degree, exhibited inadequate follow-up after resection. To delve deeper, the study suggested that individuals with a high school diploma experienced a reduced risk of morbidity and mortality, contrasting with those residing in areas lacking comparable educational advantages [52].

7.1.2 Socioeconomic burden of meningioma

Socioeconomic factors not only impact the quality of life of meningioma patients but are also influenced by meningioma itself, leading to a burden on socioeconomic conditions such as employment status. Consequently, this contributes to inequity and disparity in HRQoL outcomes. To be more specific, patients diagnosed with meningioma during their working years may encounter challenges that cause a decline in their quality of life, including job loss and concerns about financial stability (**Figure 1**) [40]. Overall, to gain a deeper understanding and effectively address the challenges posed by the socioeconomic burden in meningioma, there remains a crucial need for prospective studies that thoroughly investigate the associations between socioeconomic factors and HRQoL.

7.2 Healthcare factors

Another significant factor influencing HRQoL outcomes is the variation in healthcare facilities and levels of care that patients may access. Patients can experience distinct advantages based on the healthcare setting in which they receive treatment. For instance, survival rate is considered a benefit for patients with benign meningiomas who undergo surgery at academic medical centers [53].

These findings highlight a survival advantage for individuals managed within academic and research-focused programs, particularly when compared to community cancer programs. This advantage could potentially stem from a higher proportion of patients undergoing definitive initial treatment as opposed to observation, which is more prevalent in academic and research programs as compared to community-based cancer programs [53].

7.3 Demographic factors

Apart from socioeconomic and healthcare factors, demographic characteristics such as race and sex can also exert effects on HRQoL outcomes. In terms of race, Asian patients exhibit a decreased risk of death compared to white patients, whereas black patients tend to have an elevated risk of death, according to univariate analysis. Numerous studies have reported black race as a negative predictor of outcomes [54, 55]. However, when considering a stratified multivariate model that takes multiple comparisons into account, race does not demonstrate any significant association with patient outcomes. This suggests that other predictive factors likely contribute to the observed racial disparities in patient outcomes [51].

Similarly, the impacts of gender on the deterioration of HRQoL present varying results across different investigations. To illustrate, in one study, it was observed that female patients had a decreased risk of mortality in comparison to male patients. An analysis involving 12,284 patients from the Surveillance, Epidemiology, and End Results (SEER) database documented a reduced risk of death among female patients with meningiomas [54]. This trend was also observed in research by Achey et al., who identified a survival advantage for females in non-malignant meningiomas using data from the Central Brain Tumor Registry of the United States [55]. On the other hand, there are studies that did not reveal noteworthy disparities in HRQoL outcomes based on gender [53].

8. Conclusion

Meningiomas stand as the most common type of primary brain tumor in adults, with the majority of them remaining asymptomatic. Interestingly, even minimally symptomatic patients can experience impaired well-being and HRQoL compared to healthy individuals. In detail, various domains of HRQoL can be affected by meningioma, including physical functioning, neurocognitive and psychosocial functioning,

As a result of advancements in therapeutic approaches and subsequent rise in life expectancy, the focus of treatment purposes has been shifted from only striving for survival to prioritizing patient performance and HRQoL. To evaluate HRQoL, various self-assessment questionnaires have been developed for patients to report their own experiences and perceptions of HRQoL. However, they could not specifically address meningioma-related issues. Therefore, meningioma-specific concerns may not be considered and met thoroughly by these instruments [10].

To estimate HRQoL, there are various risk factors, such as histologic grade, location, size and recurrence of tumor, and burden of seizure contributing to worse HRQoL outcomes in short and long time. In the long run, some patients are likely to be involved in unemployment and, consequently financial issues, which may have detrimental effects on their HRQoL. To address this challenge, it would be essential to benefit from novel technology (AI), predict patients' perspective HRQoL, allocate supportive care services, and implement rehabilitation systems tailored to their specific needs.

Regarding treatment, although therapeutic interventions such as surgery and radiotherapy can improve seizure control and reduce reliance on antiepileptic drugs, HRQoL scores may still remain stabilized or diminished in some patients. We hope that researchers will develop alternative therapeutic options that hold the potential to improve HRQoL further compared to existing therapies.

Beyond treatment, it is imperative to address the issue of equitable care outcomes for meningioma patients and address the disparities in HRQoL outcomes stemming from socioeconomic, healthcare, and demographic factors. Efforts to bridge these gaps and ensure equality in HRQoL outcomes are of paramount importance.

Overall, enhancing HRQoL outcomes for meningioma patients requires a comprehensive approach that addresses both medical and psychosocial factors derived from the tumor and focuses on interactive communication for effective monitoring of their HRQoL, which helps to optimize patient well-being and functional outcomes. These tools (PROMs) aid clinicians in understanding patients' limitations and dependency levels and allow for monitoring outcome, and assessing postoperative changes in the quality of life. Making informed treatment decisions over the long term is of paramount importance for meningioma patients, as it ensures practical and effective management of their condition.

Conflict of interest

The authors declare no conflict of interest.

Author details

Mohsen Merati[1], Fateme Montazeri[2], Farnam Mohebi[3]*, Hannaneh Kabir[4] and Hamidreza Komaki[5]

1 Division of Gastroenterology, Department of Medicine, University of California, San Francisco, California, United States of America

2 Department of Ophthalmology and Vision Sciences, University of California, Davis, Sacramento, California, United States of America

3 Hass Hall, University of California at Berkeley, California, United States of America

4 Department of Bioengineering, University of California at Berkeley, California, United States of America

5 Khoury College of Computer Sciences, Northeastern University, San Francisco, California, United States of America

*Address all correspondence to: farnam.mohebi@gmail.com

References

[1] Haider S, Taphoorn MJ, Drummond KJ, Walbert T. Health-related quality of life in meningioma. Neuro-Oncology Advances. 2021;**3**(1):vdab089

[2] Whittle IR, Smith C, Navoo P, Collie D. Meningiomas. The Lancet. 2004;**363**(9420):1535-1543

[3] van Alkemade H et al. Impaired survival and long-term neurological problems in benign meningioma. Neuro-Oncology. 2012;**14**(5):658-666

[4] Lisowski D et al. Health-related quality of life and clinical outcome after radiotherapy of patients with intracranial meningioma. Scientific Reports. 2022;**12**(1):19730

[5] Sitlinger A, Zafar SY. Health-related quality of life: The impact on morbidity and mortality. Surgical Oncology Clinics of North America. 2018;**27**(4):675-684

[6] Corniola MV, Meling TR. Functional outcome and quality of life after meningioma surgery: A systematic review. Acta Neurologica Scandinavica. 2021;**143**(5):467-474

[7] Slevin ML et al. Who should measure quality of life, the doctor or the patient? British Journal of Cancer. 1988;**57**(1):109-112

[8] Schiestel C, Ryan D. Quality of life in patients with meningiomas: The true meaning of "benign". Frontiers in Bioscience-Elite. 2009;**1**(2):488-493

[9] Salas M et al. Validated instruments of quality of life (QOL) in patients with acute myeloid leukemia (AML) and other cancers. Frontiers in Pharmacology. 2020;**11**:1109

[10] Näslund O et al. Indications and outcome in surgically treated asymptomatic meningiomas: A single-center case-control study. Acta Neurochirurgica. 2020;**162**:2155-2163

[11] Zamanipoor Najafabadi AH et al. Determinants and predictors for the long-term disease burden of intracranial meningioma patients. Journal of Neuro-Oncology. 2021;**151**:201-210

[12] Zamanipoor Najafabadi AH et al. Impaired health-related quality of life in meningioma patients—A systematic review. Neuro-Oncology. 2017;**19**(7):897-907

[13] Zamanipoor Najafabadi AH et al. Unmet needs and recommendations to improve meningioma care through patient, partner, and health care provider input: A mixed-method study. Neuro-Oncology Practice. 2020;**7**(2):239-248

[14] Schiavolin S, Mariniello A, Broggi M, DiMeco F, Ferroli P, Leonardi M. Preoperative nonmedical predictors of functional impairment after brain tumor surgery. Supportive Care in Cancer: Official Journal of the Multinational Association of Supportive Care in Cancer. 2022;**30**(4):3441-3450. DOI: 10.1007/s00520-021-06732-6

[15] Mathiesen T et al. Effects of using combined transpetrosal surgical approaches to treat petroclival meningiomas. Neurosurgery. 2008;**62**(6):SHC1213-SHC1223

[16] Mohsenipour I et al. Quality of life in patients after meningioma resection. Acta Neurochirurgica. 2001;**143**:547-553

[17] Powell T, Ekin-Wood A, Collin C. Post-traumatic growth after head injury:

A long-term follow-up. Brain Injury. 2007;**21**(1):31-38

[18] Sprangers MA, Schwartz CE. Integrating response shift into health-related quality of life research: A theoretical model. Social Science & Medicine. 1999;**48**(11):1507-1515

[19] Van Nieuwenhuizen D et al. Neurocognitive functioning and health-related quality of life in patients with radiologically suspected meningiomas. Journal of Neuro-Oncology. 2013;**113**:433-440

[20] Waagemans ML et al. Long-term impact of cognitive deficits and epilepsy on quality of life in patients with low-grade meningiomas. Neurosurgery. 2011;**69**(1):72-79

[21] Meling TR, Da Broi M, Scheie D, Helseth E. Meningiomas: skull base versus non-skull base. Neurosurgical Review. 2019;**42**:163-173

[22] Karsy M et al. EQ-5D quality-of-life analysis and cost-effectiveness after skull base meningioma resection. Neurosurgery. 2019;**85**(3):E543-E552

[23] Tucha O et al. Preoperative and postoperative cognitive functioning in patients with frontal meningiomas. Journal of Neurosurgery. 2003;**98**(1):21-31

[24] Meskal I et al. Cognitive improvement in meningioma patients after surgery: Clinical relevance of computerized testing. Journal of Neuro-Oncology. 2015;**121**:617-625

[25] Bunevicius A et al. Predictors of health-related quality of life in neurosurgical brain tumor patients: Focus on patient-centered perspective. Acta Neurochirurgica. 2014;**156**: 367-374

[26] Eaton WW et al. Population-based study of first onset and chronicity in major depressive disorder. Archives of General Psychiatry. 2008;**65**(5):513-520

[27] Ghandour F et al. Presenting psychiatric and neurological symptoms and signs of brain tumors before diagnosis: A systematic review. Brain Sciences. 2021;**11**(3):301

[28] Hussin S, Yusoff SSM, Zin FM. Frontal meningioma with psychiatric symptoms. Journal of Family Medicine and Primary Care. 2018;7(1):252

[29] Das S, Prasad S, Reddy B. Severe depression with psychosis as a primary psychiatric manifestation in a patient with frontal meningioma. Psychiatry Research Case Reports. 2022;**1**(2):100015

[30] Schwartz AC, Afejuku A, Garlow SJ. Bifrontal meningioma presenting as postpartum depression with psychotic features. Psychosomatics. 2013;**2**(54):187-191

[31] Malhi G, Lagopoulos J. Making sense of neuroimaging in psychiatry. Acta Psychiatrica Scandinavica. 2008;**117**(2):100-117

[32] Wu A et al. Presenting symptoms and prognostic factors for symptomatic outcomes following resection of meningioma. World Neurosurgery. 2018;**111**:e149-e159

[33] Englot DJ et al. Seizures in supratentorial meningioma: A systematic review and meta-analysis. Journal of Neurosurgery. 2016;**124**(6):1552-1561

[34] Barrash J et al. Acquired personality disturbances after meningioma resection are strongly associated with impaired quality of life. Neurosurgery. 2020;**87**(2):276

[35] Jiang B, Quinones-Hinojosa A. Treatment of epileptic seizures in brain tumors: A critical review-commentary. Neurosurgical Review. 2014;**37**(3):388

[36] Elbadry Ahmed R, Tang H, Asemota A, Huang L, Boling W, Bannout F. Meningioma related epilepsy-pathophysiology, pre/postoperative seizures predicators and treatment. Frontiers in Oncology. 2022;**12**:905976. Published 2022 Jul 4. DOI: 10.3389/fonc.2022.905976

[37] Hess K et al. Brain invasion and the risk of seizures in patients with meningioma. Journal of Neurosurgery. 2018;**130**(3):789-796

[38] DeGeorge EG et al. Effects of age of onset and medication on cognitive performance and quality of life in patients with epilepsy. Epilepsy & Behavior. 2021;**121**:108008

[39] Jakola AS, Gulati M, Gulati S, Solheim O. The influence of surgery on quality of life in patients with intracranial meningiomas: A prospective study. Journal of Neuro-Oncology. 2012;**110**:137-144

[40] Wirsching H-G, Morel C, Roth P, Weller M. Socioeconomic burden and quality of life in meningioma patients. Quality of Life Research. 2020;**29**:1801-1808

[41] Miao Y et al. A multivariate analysis of prognostic factors for health-related quality of life in patients with surgically managed meningioma. Journal of Clinical Neuroscience. 2010;**17**(4):446-449

[42] Ferroli P et al. Predicting functional impairment in brain tumor surgery: The big five and the Milan complexity scale. Neurosurgical Focus. 2015;**39**(6):E14

[43] Lubgan D et al. Stereotactic radiotherapy as primary definitive or postoperative treatment of intracranial meningioma of WHO grade II and III leads to better disease control than stereotactic radiotherapy of recurrent meningioma. Journal of Neuro-Oncology. 2017;**134**:407-416

[44] Pollock BE, Stafford SL. Results of stereotactic radiosurgery for patients with imaging defined cavernous sinus meningiomas. International Journal of Radiation Oncology, Biology, Physics. 2005;**62**(5):1427-1431

[45] Meskal I, Gehring K, Rutten G-JM, Sitskoorn MM. Cognitive functioning in meningioma patients: A systematic review. Journal of Neuro-Oncology. 2016;**128**:195-205

[46] van Nieuwenhuizen D et al. Differential effect of surgery and radiotherapy on neurocognitive functioning and health-related quality of life in WHO grade I meningioma patients. Journal of Neuro-Oncology. 2007;**84**:271-278

[47] Nassiri F et al. Life after surgical resection of a meningioma: A prospective cross-sectional study evaluating health-related quality of life. Neuro-Oncology. 2019;**21**(Supplement_1):i32-i43

[48] Yang Z et al. Machine learning and statistical prediction of patient quality-of-life after prostate radiation therapy. Computers in Biology and Medicine. 2021;**129**:104127

[49] Kumar S et al. PrediQt-cx: Post treatment health related quality of life prediction model for cervical cancer patients. PLoS One. 2014;**9**(2):e89851

[50] Karri R, Chen Y-PP, Drummond KJ. Using machine learning to predict health-related quality of life outcomes

in patients with low grade glioma, meningioma, and acoustic neuroma. PLoS One. 2022;**17**(5):e0267931

[51] Yang AI, Mensah-Brown KG, Rinehart C, et al. Inequalities in meningioma survival: Results from the national cancer database. Cureus. 2020;**12**(3):e7304. Published 2020 Mar 18. DOI: 10.7759/cureus.7304

[52] Nayeri A, Brinson PR, Weaver KD, Thompson RC, Chambless LB. Factors associated with low socioeconomic status predict poor postoperative follow-up after meningioma resection. Journal of Neurological Surgery Part B: Skull Base. 2016;**77**(3):226-230. DOI: 10.1055/s-0035-1566122

[53] McKee SP et al. Intracranial meningioma surgery: Value-based care determinants in New York state, 1995-2015. World Neurosurgery. 2018;**118**:e731-e744

[54] Cahill KS, Claus EB. Treatment and survival of patients with nonmalignant intracranial meningioma: Results from the surveillance, epidemiology, and end results program of the National Cancer Institute. Journal of Neurosurgery. 2011;**115**(2):259-267

[55] Achey RL et al. Nonmalignant and malignant meningioma incidence and survival in the elderly, 2005-2015, using the central brain tumor registry of the United States. Neuro-Oncology. 2019;**21**(3):380-391

Chapter 4

Radiosurgery for Intracranial Meningiomas

Gustavo Zomosa, Claudio Lühr, Francisco Bova, Lucas González-Johnson, Catalina Rojas-Solé, Lene Troncoso, Gonzalo Miranda and José Lorenzoni

Abstract

The classical definition of stereotactic radiosurgery (SRS) involves administering a high dose of radiation within a limited treatment area. More recently, it has also encompassed the concept of hypofractionated radiosurgery, which involves delivering radiation over up to five treatment sessions. Intracranial meningiomas (IM) are commonly encountered primary brain tumors. Currently, there has been a rise in the number of asymptomatic individuals with IM, who subsequently require treatment due to the development and onset of symptoms. Small and medium-sized IM treatment standard options encompass radical surgery; however, this may not always be feasible due to surgical risks and patient preferences. In contrast, SRS stands out as an effective tool for managing tumor growth and alleviating symptoms. It is an outpatient procedure that eliminates the need for general anesthesia and extensive postoperative care. This holds particular significance in countries with long surgical waitlists, providing a cost-effective and low complication alternative. Furthermore, SRS plays a crucial role not only in grade I IM but also in addressing some cases of recurrent and residual grade II and even grade III IM. It also has a place in the management of radiation-induced meningioma.

Keywords: meningioma, radiosurgery, gamma knife radiosurgery, stereotactic radiosurgery, outcomes

1. Introduction

Intracranial meningiomas (IM) represent the most prevalent primary central nervous system (CNS) tumors in adults, with an incidence rate ranging from 8.58 to 9.15 cases per 100,000 individuals. They account for 55% of nonmalignant brain tumors within the general population of the United States [1, 2]. While most meningiomas are typically benign, their presence within the CNS can lead to significant morbidity or even mortality, thereby profoundly impacting both patient survival and quality of life. Meningiomas can originate from various locations within the dura mater, most frequently occurring within the skull and sites of dural reflection (falx cerebri, tentorium cerebelli, venous sinuses) [3].

IntechOpen

Recognized risk factors for this condition include age > 65 years, female (double age-adjusted) [2], African-American race, exposure to ionizing radiation, and genetic factors as neurofibromatosis type II (NFII) [1]. According to studies, males are more likely to be higher grade II and III [4–6].

It is believed that these tumors originate from meningoendothelial cells within the arachnoid cap. In a prospective magnetic resonance imaging (MRI) study involving 5800 participants, incidental IM was estimated to occur in approximately 2.5% of cases [7]. These tumors exhibit a mean annual growth rate of 1 cm^3, and about 11% of incidentally asymptomatic meningiomas will demonstrate growth, potentially causing symptoms if the growth rate exceeds 2.1 cm^3 per year and the tumor size surpasses 4 cm in diameter [8, 9].

Meningiomas are predominantly benign (WHO grade I), accounting for 80–85% of cases, while a smaller but growing proportion in recent years is classified as atypical (WHO grade II), ranging from 15–18%. A minority of cases are categorized as anaplastic (WHO grade III), constituting 1-3% of cases [10].

The most common locations for IM are supratentorial, occurring in 40–60% of cases [11]. They can be further classified into skull base and non-skull base tumors, with subclassification based on the location of dural attachment [4]. In individuals with neurofibromatosis type II (NFII), it is possible to develop multiple meningiomas [12].

Radiosurgery, as originally described by Leksell (and later developing Gamma Knife (GK)), involves the precise delivery of a single high dose of radiation to a small and well-defined target volume [13]. This precision is achieved through the utilization of multiple radiation beams that converge on the target with the full therapeutic dose confined to the area where all these beams overlap. In contrast, nontarget areas receive substantially smaller doses from just one or a limited number of the radiation beams, with a rapid reduction in dose beyond the target to spare the surrounding healthy tissue. To enhance the accuracy of radiation targeting and delivery, an external localization system is employed [13].

One crucial requirement for successful stereotactic radiosurgery (SRS) is that the radiation target must be adequately separated from normal tissues that could be harmed by the high dose administered in a single treatment session. This technique has emerged as an effective alternative for managing selected small and medium IM [1].

In cases involving larger tumors, an alternative approach is hypofractionated radiosurgery (HSRS), which will be reviewed later.

The suggested mechanisms for restraining tumor growth involve a combination of impairment of the tumor cells' ability to replicate and the induction of vascular hyalinization, leading to fibrosis and necrosis. Biopsies from patients with WHO grade I IM who underwent SRS treatment revealed distinct findings in enhanced and non-enhanced regions. In enhanced areas, there was evidence of inflammation, demyelination, and the development of cystic changes. Meanwhile, in non-enhanced areas, coagulative necrosis, edema, vasculopathy, and reactive astrocytosis were observed (**Figure 1**) [14].

The therapeutic approach relies on a combination of factors, including the presence of symptoms, the size of the tumor, and its location. When dealing with a symptomatic tumor that is actively growing and causing mass effect, especially if it is in an accessible location, surgical resection becomes the recommended course of action. However, if complete and safe tumor removal is not achievable, as is often the case with tumors located at the skull base, then alternative treatments may be considered. For small remaining growing tumors, radiosurgery can be employed, while fractionated radiotherapy is a viable option for larger ones [1].

According to EANO guidelines, in the case of incidental asymptomatic suspected intracranial meningiomas, it is advisable to conduct annual MRI scans over a 5-year

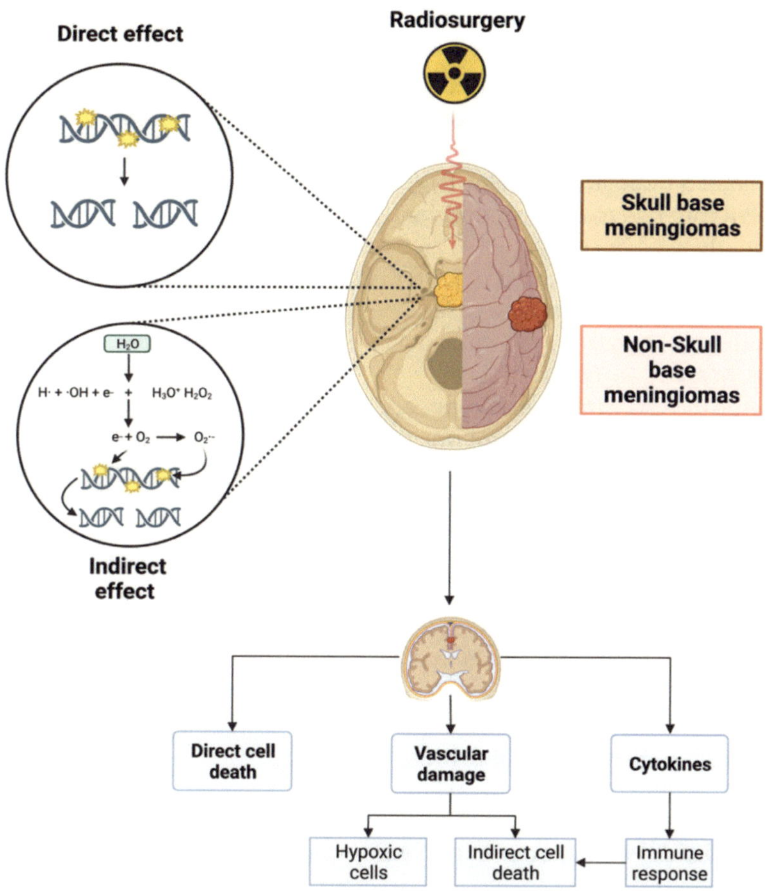

Figure 1.
Radiosurgery mechanism of action. Figure created with Biorender.com.

period. This monitoring is crucial for observing any growth in the tumor or the development of symptoms that may warrant treatment. It is also essential to remain vigilant for potential cognitive deficits that could be easily overlooked during this surveillance process [15].

The primary reasons to consider SRS for IM include cases where the tumor is either asymptomatic or causing minimal symptoms, particularly when there is documented tumor growth or the potential for symptom development [12]. Additionally, SRS is a viable option in situations where the surgical risks are prohibitively high or when it aligns with the patient's preferences. Furthermore, SRS can be considered for cases of recurrence of small to moderate size following a gross total resection (GTR) [1, 12]. An article from a Swedish group showed that in patients with deliberated non-radical IM surgery (Simpson grade IV) associated with a combined adjuvant-GK radiosurgery treatment allowed return to a low recurrence rate of 10% (similar to Simpson grade I) in tumors with a low proliferative index (direct GK SRS after tailored microsurgical resection Simpson IV gamma) [16]. An alternative approach known as staged SRS has been documented for larger tumors, typically ranging from 20 to 30 cm^3 in size. These sizable tumors are divided into several manageable portions, each of which can be treated at intervals spanning months [17].

2. SRS technique

Stereotactic radiosurgery can be conducted in two primary ways. The classic approach involves a single session, during which a frame is securely fixed in place under local anesthesia, ensuring submillimeter precision. Alternatively, there is hypofractionated radiosurgery (HSRS) (i.e., Cyberknife and GK Icon), which divides the treatment into two to five fractions and a dose per fraction ≥5 Gy. In HSRS, the most frequently used dose regimen is 25 Gy delivered over five fractions [18]. This irradiation technique can be used in larger tumors or those near organs at risk (OAR). It is important to note that in such cases, specific dose constraints are adhered to the maximum allowable dose for the optic nerve is <8 Gy, for the brainstem it is <12 Gy, and for the cochlea it is <4 Gy [12].

In SRS, the most favorable outcomes are typically observed in tumors with a diameter of less than 3 cm and a volume smaller than 10 cm^3 [1]. For HSRS, which is a frameless technique utilizing a thermoplastic mask, precision is paramount. Various systems, such as online navigation, as exemplified by the GK Icon, are employed to ensure the accuracy of the procedure [1, 12].

Single-session SRS and HSRS use thin slide pre/post-contrast MRI fused with a CT scan obtained with a stereotactic frame for treatment planning [1]. The treatment volume should include the entire tumor and nodular thickened dura [1]. The usual prescription dose for IM is 12–16 Gy to the tumor margin at the 50% isodose [12]. Single-session SRS with prescription dose of at least 14 Gy is associated with a 5-year control rate of ≥90% for benign meningiomas [18, 19]. Dose greater than 16 Gy is associated with a higher rate of SRS-induced edema [20].

3. General clinical outcomes with SRS

In 2008, the Pittsburg experience reported 1045 IM with a tumor control rate of 97% and 95% at 5 and 10 years in patients who underwent primary SRS. A total of 49% of these patients underwent a prior resection with a mean treated volume of 7.4 cm^3, and the control rate was 93% at 5 years and 91% at 10 years. The symptom control was 93% in primary and 91% in adjuvant patients. The overall morbidity was 7.7% and symptomatic but transient imaging changes were present in 4% of patients [21]. The tumor control rate was poorer for WHO grade II (50%) and grade III (17%) [22].

The European multicenter study of Santacroce et al. involved the examination of 4566 patients with IM of an average volume of 4.8 cm^3 and an average treatment margin dose (MD) of 14 Gy. Their results revealed a progression-free survival (PFS) rate of 95.2% at the 5-year and 88.6% at the 10-year. Notably, the study demonstrated a reduction in tumor volume by 58%, stability in 34.5%, and an increase in 7.5% of cases. The study documented enduring morbidity at a rate of 6.6%, with a concomitant disability incidence of 1.2% [23].

The International SRS Society published a meta-analysis with 3750 non-cavernous sinus IM from 27 studies (1964–2018) with an average volume of 5.6 cm^3 for single-dose treatment with an average MD of 14 Gy and 6.4 cm^3 for HSRS treated with 25 Gy in five fractions. They reported post-SRS that neurologic deterioration was from 0% to 13.3%, with a median of 7.4% according to eight studies. The meta-analysis of 6 of these studies, suggests an overall symptom control rate of 95.1% (95% CI: 92.1–97.5%). The radiation toxicity ranged from 2.5% to 34.6% (median 8.0%) in 13 papers.

The meta-analysis of 11 of the studies, showed an overall post-SRS toxicity of 11% (95% CI: 6.4–16.5%) but with a high heterogeneity among the original studies [18].

4. IM locations specific outcomes

4.1 Non-skull base IM

4.1.1 Convexity meningioma

Convexity meningiomas are the most common location (30%); the preferred first option treatment is GTR (Simpson grade I or II) [12]. But in some patients, this is not possible, and SRS is an option for small to medium tumors. More detail is presented in **Table 1**.

4.1.2 Parasagittal and parafalcine

This is the second most common location and surgical resection may be limited by the anatomical involvement of the nearby venous sinuses, so there is a place for SRS as primary or adjuvant therapy [12]. Sheehan in 2015 from the same group reported about the factors that are associated with new or progressive edema: tumor volume greater than 10 cm^3, a higher margin dose, and absence of prior resection [26].

4.2 Skull base

Skull base meningiomas locations include clivus, petroclival, parasellar, and cerebellopontine angle (**Figure 2**).

IM location	Dose	Results	Comments	Reference
Convexity	14.2 Gy	Control rate at: • 3 years: 95% • 5 years: 86%	• Morbidity rate: 10% • Symptomatic tumoral edema: 5%.	Kondziolka et al. [24]
Parasagittal and Parafalcine	15 Gy	Control rate* at: • 3 years: 85% • 5 years: 70%	• Symptomatic tumoral edema: 8.2% • Permanent clinical sequelae: 2%	Ding et al. [25]
	10–20Gy	PFS: • 2 years: 98% • 5 years: 90%	• New peritumoral edema that progress: 14%	Sheehan et al. [26]
	12.7 Gy	Control rate at: • 5 years: 91% • 10 years: 89%	• Symptomatic tumoral edema: 3% • Symptomatic improvement: 41% • Volume reduction: 61%	Martínez-Pérez et al. [27]

**The study of Ding et al. achieved a low level of tumor control because treatment planning did not always cover the long dural tail.*

Table 1.
Non-skull base IM — Summary of findings from different studies.

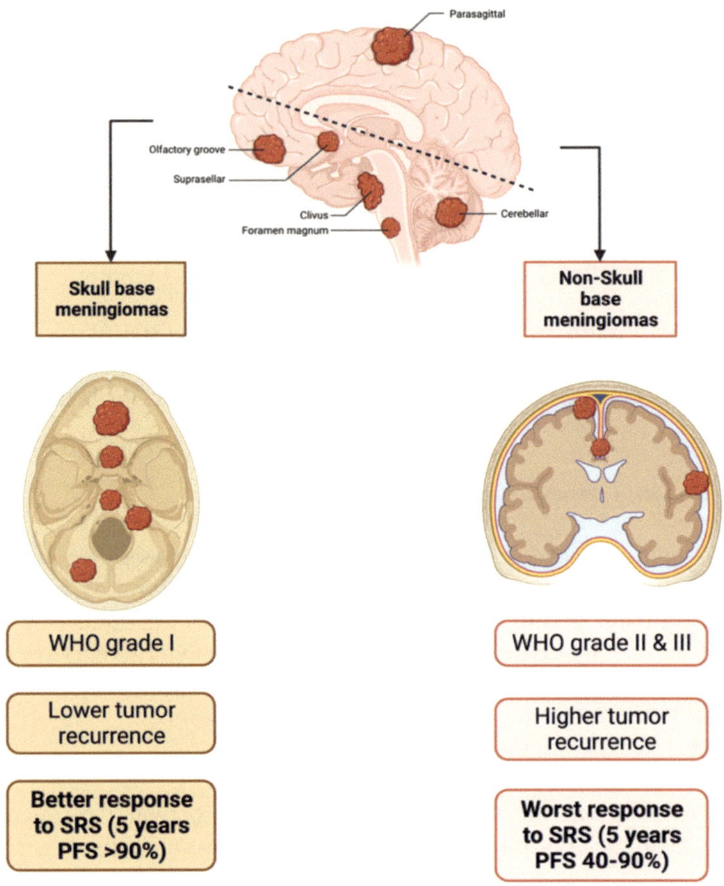

Figure 2.
Main tumor locations of IM — Skull base meningioma and non-skull base meningioma. PFS, progression-free survival; SRS, stereotactic radiosurgery. Figure created by authors using Biorrender.com.

The retrospective Austrian study from Kreil and Cols. analyzed long-term data from 200 patients with benign skull base meningioma. The median tumor volume was 6.5 cm^3 treated with median MD of 12 Gy with GK. They reported a 5- and 10-year PFS of 98.5 and 97.2%, respectively. Neurological status improved in 41.5% of cases, remained unaltered in 54%, and deteriorated in 4.5%. Of the deteriorated subgroup, the majority was transient (7 of 9 patients). Treatment failure that required reoperation was reported in 2.5% of cases [28]. The retrospective American study from Starke et al. documented 225 patients with skull base meningiomas (average pre-GK volume of 5.0 cm^3). In this cohort, with a median follow-up duration of 6.5 years, only 14% of cases exhibited an increase in tumor volume and 86% exhibited a decrease or stable tumor volume. PFS rates reported at 3-, 5- and 10-years were 99, 96, and 79% respectively. Neurological status deteriorated in only 10 and 90% remained unaltered or improved (**Table 2**) [36].

SRS for skull base IM produces excellent tumor control with low morbidity rates compared with surgery alone for asymptomatic small skull base IM, patients with high surgical risk, and as an adjuvant therapy for recurrent or residual lesions [37].

IM location	Median dose	Results	Comments	Reference
Petroclival	13 Gy	PFS rates at: • 5 years: 91% • 10 years: 86%	• Volume reduction: 46% • Symptom control: 85%	Flannery et al. [29]
	13.5 Gy	PFS rates at: • 5 years: 91–100% • 10 years: 69.6–89.9%	Tumor control: 94.3% • Less complications with primary SRS versus adjuvant therapy: 3.7% • Improve or remain unchanged of functional status	Bin Alamer et al. [30]
Cavernous sinus	14 Gy	PFS rates at: • 5 years: 86–99% • 10 years: 69–97%	• Neurological preservation rate post SRS: 80–100%	Lee et al. [31]
	13.5 Gy	PFS rates at: • 5 years: 93.4% • 10 years: 84.9% • 15 years: 81.3%	• Cranial nerve deficit improvement: 36.4%, primary SRS > adjuvant • Widening of cranial nerve deficit: 11.5% • Imaging regression: 57.8% • Tumor progression: 8.5%	Martínez-Pérez et al. [32]
Parasellar	14 Gy	Tumor control rate: • 6 Years: 91.5%	• Tumor progression: 8,5% • Direct complications related to SRS: 2.64%	Cohen-Inbar et al. [33]
Orbital	10–15 Gy	Tumor control rate: • 5 years: ≈ 90%*	• Volume reduction: 53.5% • Remain stable: 41.6% • Tumor progression: 4.7%	Xu et al. [34]
Intraventricular	14 Gy	Tumor control rate • 4 years: 100%	• Volume reduction: 55% • Transient perifocal edema: 37%	Umekawa et al. [35]

**This study included a variety of orbital tumors. The most prominent were meningiomas.*

Table 2.
Skull base IM — Summary of findings from different studies.

4.2.1 Petroclival meningiomas (PCIM)

Petroclival meningiomas arise from the upper two-thirds of the clivus with dural attachment centered on the petroclival junction and medial to the V nerve [3]. If it is possible, skull base microsurgery is the first-line choice of treatment considering that GTR is the only curative option, offering immediate relief from mass effect and decompression. However, it is often impossible to achieve a complete resection due to invasion to neurovascular structures, and it is associated with high morbidity rates from 28 to 76% and mortality from 3.7 to 17% [30]. Indeed, considering the high rates of surgical complications, SRS is a low-rate complication procedure that offers high levels of tumor control and is a valid option as an adjuvant in residual or recurrent PCIM [12].

The retrospective American study of Flannery et al. reported 168 patients with PCIM (average pre-GK volume of 6.1 cm^3) who underwent GK SRS (median marginal dose was 13 Gy). In this report, with a median follow-up of 72 months, only 10% of cases exhibited an increase in tumor volume and 90% exhibited a decrease or stable tumor volume. Symptoms and neurological status were controlled in 85% of cases. PFS rates reported at 5- and 10-years were 91 and 86%, respectively. Also, initial or further surgical resection were obviated in 98% of patients with a low risk of adverse radiation effects [29].

Bin Alamer et al. conducted a systematic review and meta-analysis, encompassing seven articles that involved 722 patients with PCIM. Neurovascular invasion to cavernous sinus, brainstem, and Meckel's cave occurred in 37, 23.9, and 21.7%, respectively. Additionally, most cases were classified as WHO grade I, constituting 97.3% of the total cases [37].

The mean tumor volume was 8.1 cm^3, and these patients received a marginal dose of 13.5 Gy. Primary SRS was administered to 61.9% of patients, achieving a tumor control rate of 94.3% with SRS complications at 3.7%. Additionally, 38.1% underwent adjuvant SRS, resulting in lower tumor control (88.2%) and higher rate of complications (10.3%).

Post SRS, symptoms improved in 28.7%, remained unchanged in 61.3%, and worsened in only 10%, while the functional status of primary SRS remained stable or improved. Tumor PFS ranged from 91 to 100% over 5 years and 69.6–89.9% over 10 years. The most common post-SRS complications included V deficit (15.1%), followed by hydrocephalus (9.3%), ataxia (8.1%), and dizziness (8.1%) [30].

In a clinical setting, a total safe resection is ideal, including debulking and decompression of the brainstem and cranial nerves, (especially in the case of large symptomatic tumors exceeding 10 cm^3). Subsequently, adjuvant SRS is recommended for any remaining post-resection PCIM to attain effective tumor control with minimal complications [38–40].

4.2.2 Cavernous sinus meningiomas (CSIM)

Cavernous sinus meningiomas represent 10% of skull base meningiomas and are the most common primary cavernous sinus tumors [41]. In general, CSIM are benign skull base tumors with low volumetric tumoral growth [11]. According to Klinger and Cols, 34–77% of patients with CSIM showed tumoral growth within 4 years [42].

Surgery for CSIM is linked with high rates of morbidity and mortality [42, 43]. Therefore, SRS is a valid option for CSIM control either as primary or as adjuvant therapy [32].

The study of Lee et al. reported 159 patients treated with GK SRS for CSIM. A total of 52% of the patients were treated as primary radiosurgery, and 98% were benign WHO grade I. After treatment, the neurological status improved in 29%, remained stable in 62%, and worsened in 6% of patients. The results reveal that 60% of patients sustained a stable tumor volume, with an increase observed in only 6% of cases. Moreover, the 5-year tumor control rate stood notably high at 96.9% among individuals who exclusively underwent SRS as their therapeutic intervention [44].

The International Stereotactic Radiosurgery Society conducted a systematic review and guideline about the treatment with SRS for benign CSIM. They analyzed 49 retrospective studies, most of them with favorable outcomes with 5- and 10-year PFS rates ranging from 86–99% and 69–97%, respectively. The post-SRS neurological preservation rate ranged from 80–100%. Based on the observed results, SRS offers a favorable benefit-risk profile. Using single-session with a marginal dose of 11-16 Gy offers a local tumor control rate of ≥ 90% at 5 years with low risk of complication. The authors recommend the use of SRS as a primary treatment option for an asymptomatic or mildly symptomatic CSIM. The study recommended to consider SRS for tumor recurrence or progression for residual tumor [31].

In a more recent systematic review and meta-analysis of Martinez-Perez et al. analyzed seven studies, comprising 645 CSIM patients with documented long-term follow-up (more than 60 months). The calculated PFS at 5, 10, and 15 years were 93.4, 84.9, and 81.3%, respectively. Most patients had no changes in cranial nerve function; the improvement of cranial nerve deficits was found in 36.4% and worsening or new onset of cranial nerve deficits was observed in only 11.5%. The imaging regression was found in 57.8%, and tumor progression was seen in 8.5% [32].

In conclusion, these studies have shown that SRS can achieve long-term tumor control in CSIM as primary and adjuvant therapy with a low rate of complications [32].

4.2.3 Parasellar meningiomas (PSIM)

Parasellar meningiomas often extend into the suprasellar, cavernous sinus, and petroclival regions, potentially involving critical neurovascular structures. In such complex scenarios, achieving total resection can be challenging and may carry significant morbidity. In such cases, SRS presents itself as a viable alternative for both primary and adjuvant therapy [12]. In a 2018, study involving 189 patients diagnosed with PSIM and a median tumor volume of 5.6 cm^3, approximately 44% of the cases underwent primary GK SRS. The findings showed a favorable tumor control rate of 91.5%, with in-field recurrences occurring at a rate of 4.2%, and out-field recurrences also at 4.2% [33]. New or worsening neurological deficits were observed in 28.5% due to tumor progression in 90.7% of patients and 9.3% due to SRS. A total of 10% involved trigeminal nerve and 9.5% optic nerve dysfunction. The early follow-up (3 years) measurements predicted long-term volume changes and tumor volume control at 10 years [33].

4.2.4 Orbital (OIM): orbital wall meningiomas and optic sheath meningiomas

Orbital IM can be divided into two groups. One group, which is implanted in orbital walls and compresses the optic nerve, which can be resected. On the other hand, the second group called optic sheath meningiomas (OSM) cannot be excised. In a series of 19 OIM implanted in orbital walls, 54% had been operated before with a mean volume of 6 cm^3 and received a median dose of 12.8 Gy. A total of 5% showed better vision, 75% were unchanged, and 20% were blind in that eye [45]. A total of 20% suffered transient neuropathic orbital pain. OSM represents 2% of the orbital tumors [46, 47], and untreated, compression of the optic nerve leads to amaurosis in the affected eye. They may be primary or secondary from the extra-orbital meninges and if visual impairment occurs then active therapy is indicated also because of the risk of contralateral involvement, especially in secondary origin. Surgery is only indicated in poor visual function, proptosis, intracranial extension, or contralateral growth [47, 48]. Then as Turbin et al. [49] concluded that radiation therapy was the better therapy, and more recently hypofractionated GK SRS has been reported as the therapy of choice [50, 51].

4.2.5 Intraventricular meningiomas (IVM)

Meningiomas located within the ventricles are infrequent, accounting for approximately 0.3–5% of all IM [52].

Despite recent advancements in surgical techniques, such as neuroendoscopy, the management of intraventricular meningiomas (IVM) remains challenging due to their deep-seated location and proximity to critical neural tracts. This challenging surgical scenario is associated with a notably high complication rate of approximately 33% and a mortality rate of about 1.6% [52–54]. There are few studies about SRS in IVM, in which Umekawa reported 12 patients treated with SRS GK with 14 Gy as an MD [35]. The tumor volume decreased in 58% of cases, and an additional 48% remained stable. Consequently, effective tumor control was achieved in 100% of the tumors. As adverse radiation effects (ARE) transient perifocal edema was reported in 33% of cases. Other studies report that salvage SRS for progressive recurrent tumors failed in 67% [55, 56] but better results were obtained with upfront SRS [19]. Also, ARE was reported in 28–50% of cases and being symptomatic between 5-43% [57]. The risk of symptomatic signal MRI change was older age, larger tumor volume, higher dose, presence of pre-SRS edema, and primary SRS [57, 58]. Hence, SRS emerges as a valuable approach for achieving tumor control in IVM while preserving functional anatomy, particularly in cases where there is no significant symptomatic risk, and it is associated with minimal adverse effects.

5. SRS for IM WHO grade II and III

Biopsies from WHO grade II IM show focal necrosis with 4–10 mitosis/10 HPS and brain invasion. WHO grade III or anaplastic meningioma biopsies show marked elevation of mitotic activity, harbor a TERT promoter mutation, and homozygous detection of CDKN2A/CDKN2B [59]. The management for both grades II and III includes maximal safe resection and commonly external beam radiation therapy (EBRT) after subtotal resection (STR) to reduce the incidence of tumor recurrence [60–63].

The role of radiosurgery for WHO grade II and III and recurrent tumors is more controversial due to the suboptimal tumor control rates in some series and the need to treat the entire surgical bed in addition to gross disease, which is not often feasible with SRS [64]. However, several retrospective studies have reported acceptable local control with margin doses of 12–20 Gy [65–67].

More recently SRS has been performed as an alternative for EBRT as adjuvant treatment or for recurrence in patients that have already been irradiated [68]. Pollock reported 54 patients in Mayo Clinic with WHO grade II and III meningioma, which included four with radiation-induced meningioma [68]. The median volume was 14.6 cm^3, and the median tumor margin dose was 15 Gy. Post SRS showed tumor progression in 30% of patients, nine patients needed repeated SRS, six required tumor resection, and three repeated EBRT. The PFS at 1 year was 76% and 5 years was 40%. Multivariate analysis showed that failure of previous EBRT was a negative predictor of PFS. The incidence of radiation-induced complications (RIC) was 21% at 1 year and 23% at 5 years. A total of 18 patients had major complications.

These results may be discussed that the medium margin dose that may be needed to control grade II and grade III tumors but is not always possible because they are large tumors (median 14.6 cm^3), and the fact that patients have undergone previous EBRT. Also, the fact that most of the tumor series were supratentorial with a superior rate of this complication. Another issue is to recommend SRS to those patients that have a nodular recurrence away from critical structures (ARO) after GTR in grade II tumors. But if the recurrence is diffuse in contact with optic pathways, then EBRT must be recommended. Other institutions as the University of Virginia have similar results, and they recommend adjuvant therapy depending on the residual tumor if it is medium or small SRS and EBRT for large residual volume or close to OAR. For large recurrences, they prefer repeated surgical resections, but if it is not possible, they recommend salvage SRS for focal tumors or fractionated radiation therapy for larger recurrences or widespread disease. Also, systemic therapy as bevacizumab may be considered [69].

Based on previous evidence suggests that radiation-induced immunogenic cell death increases antigen presentation and activation of immune cells, and in combination with immune checkpoint inhibitors, subverts the immunosuppressive tumor microenvironment (abscopal effect). There is great interest in combined treatments of immune checkpoint inhibitors plus radiosurgery for recurrent or grade II/III meningioma; two ongoing clinical trials are testing SRS plus Pembrolizumab (NCT04659811) or with Nivolumab Plus or Minus Ipilimumab (NCT03604978) [70, 71].

6. SRS for treatment of radiation-induced meningioma

Radiation-induced meningioma (RIM) is a late adverse effect of cranial irradiation from pediatric malignancies [72], and they must satisfy the Cahan criteria [73]. RIMs are distinguished by specific criteria: (a) the lesion must manifest within the previously irradiated field, (b) it should emerge after a reasonable time interval following the initial therapy, (c) it must exhibit radiological and/or histological differences from the preceding neoplasm, and (d) the patient must not possess a genetic predisposition to tumor development. Notably, RIMs differ from sporadic meningioma, as they often feature histological atypia, can appear at multiple locations, posing challenges for resection and local control, and generally carry a less favorable prognosis [74]. A recent multi-institutional study from 12 institutions participating in the International Radiosurgery Research Foundation reported 52 patients treated with 60 GK SRS for histological or radiological suspected WHO grade I RIMS. The initial age at cranial irradiation was 5.5 years, and the age at SRS for RIMs was 39 years. The most common reasons for RIM were leukemia (21%) and medulloblastoma (17%). There were 39 multiple RIMs, and the mean target volume was 8.61 ± 7.5 cm^3, and volume of >5 cm^3 predicted progression. The medium prescription dose was 14 Gy. RIM progressed in 17% of patients at a median duration of 30 months after SRS. PFS at 5 years was 83%. A total of 14% of patients developed new neurological symptoms or experienced complications post SRS from 1 to 72 months after SRS. Increased risk of progression was age, volume > 5 cm^3, and multiple lesions [74].

Another study from Australia and Canada [75] reported 37 patients with 72 lesions, 62 were WHO grade I or radiologically diagnosed, six were grade II, and 4 grade III. Median volume was 2.13 cm^3 a median margin dose was 13 Gy with SRS GK single-fraction treatment. Local control at 88.6% at 5 years and for grade II and

III was 40% at 5 years. Post-SRS edema was developed in 23.6% of lesions and was symptomatic in 16.7%. As a general conclusion SRS is an effective option for certain patients such as poor surgical candidates or difficult surgical access with WHO grade I RIMs to achieve local control with acceptable safety profile and to those who progress after surgery as salvage therapy.

7. Hypofractionated radiosurgery (hypo SRS)

Hypofractionated radiosurgery represents a synergistic amalgamation of the favorable attributes inherent in SRS and the fractional administration of radiotherapy, thereby affording an expanded therapeutic domain while preserving the inherent attributes of precise targeting and conformal dosage dispersion. Additionally, a strategically planned application of this modality is discerned in cases following optic nerve decompression with residual tumor, thereby underscoring its nuanced clinical utility in select indications. Recently a prospective phase two trial was reported with 178 patients with large or critically located radiological (51%) or histological WHO grade I IM [76]. All patients were aged > 18, and Karnofsky performance status was > 70. Critical structures were optic nerve, chiasm, cavernous sinus, and brain stem. Local control was defined as complete response disappearance, partial as reduction of >20%, stable no change, or reduction <20% of tumor volume. The SRS mean dose was 25 Gy in five fractions with CyberKnife. The locations were skull base (87%), falco-tentorial (14.8%), and supratentorial (6.4%), and mean tumor volume was 14 cm^3. A total of 30% were asymptomatic and 70% presented one or more nerve dysfunction. Toxicity was 12.7% and the main events were V numbness and visual impairment. Radiation-induced optic neuropathy was observed in 5%, especially in patients with severe visual impairment before Hypo SRS. Local control was 97% at 5 years and 95% at 10 years, and partial response was achieved at 5% and stable at 45%. Only seven patients (5%) showed progression, three required surgery, and one biopsy showed an atypical meningioma grade II. In these patients, three died of progression and one of meningiomatosis progression. In 6% of asymptomatic patients, a pseudoprogression disease was observed with transient increase in tumor volume in the first 2 years after irradiation but with later tumor reduction. In conclusion, Hypo SRS is a good therapy for large IM and or for those located near OAR with good local control and low morbidity for WHO grade I IM.

8. Local experience with meningioma GK SRS treatment

Here, we present a retrospective small case series of patients with suspected IM treated with GK SRS at a Chilean radiosurgery center.

8.1 Materials and methods

8.1.1 Patient population

This is a retrospective, single-center study involving consecutive patients managed with GKRS for IM from 2011 to 2023. All data were collected in a prospective registry from the clinical patients records and then analyzed retrospectively.

201 patients who received SRS for meningioma at Centro Gamma Knife Chile during 2011-2023 were retrospectively identified. From this consecutive cohort, only 43 patients were selected for further analyses that had macroscopic tumors on baseline MRI, and additional post-SRS follow-up MRI with volumetric calculation. Irradiation treatment scheme had been recommended by experts in neurosurgery.

Data collected included patient demographics, tumor location, radiological features prior to GKRS, and at the last follow-up procedural details (e.g., radiation doses).

8.2 Radiation therapy: radiosurgical technique and gamma knife parameters

In the procedure room and under local anesthesia, patients underwent placement of a Leksell stereotactic frame. Stereotactic brain CT scanning was then obtained and fused with the preoperative, thin slice (1 mm) axial, and coronal pre- and post-contrast administration brain MRI for treatment planning. The co-registered CT and MRI images were fused in the Leksell Gamma Plan. The radiosurgical plan was formulated by the treating neurosurgeon in conjunction with a medical physicist. All patients were treated in an ambulatory setting with single-session SRS using the Leksell Gamma Knife 4C (Elekta Instruments AB). A medial marginal dose of 12.8 Gy (range from 12 to 15 Gy) was delivered in a single session with a median prescription isodose line of 48.3% (range from 35 to 60%).

8.3 Clinical and radiological follow-up

Routine clinical and radiologic follow-up was obtained at approximately 6-month intervals following GKRS. At follow-up evaluations, patients underwent a clinical examination, and new neurologic deficits were recorded. Brain MRI studies were reviewed and tumor response to GKRS was evaluated by the treating neurosurgeon (**Figures 3** and **4**).

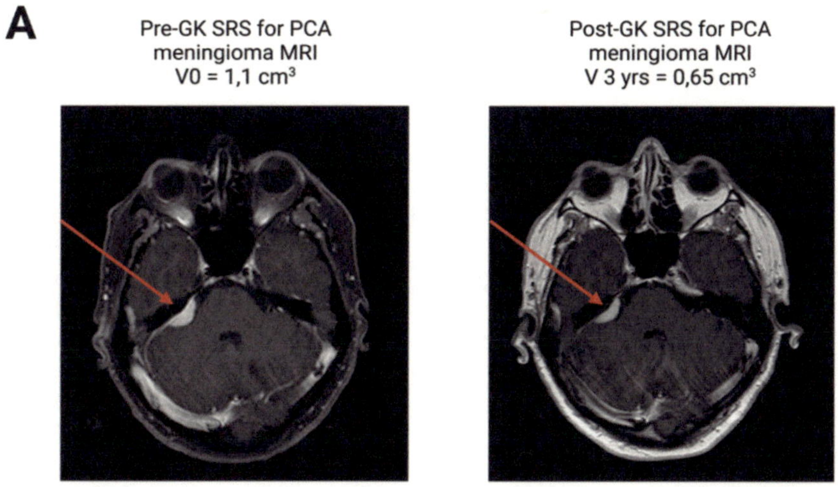

Figure 3.
A 45-year-old female with a pontocerebellar angle meningioma. She was treated in may 2012 with GK SRS 13 Gy, 55% isodose. At 3 years follow-up, there was a significant tumor volume reduction (41% tumor reduction – Minor response according to RANO) [77].

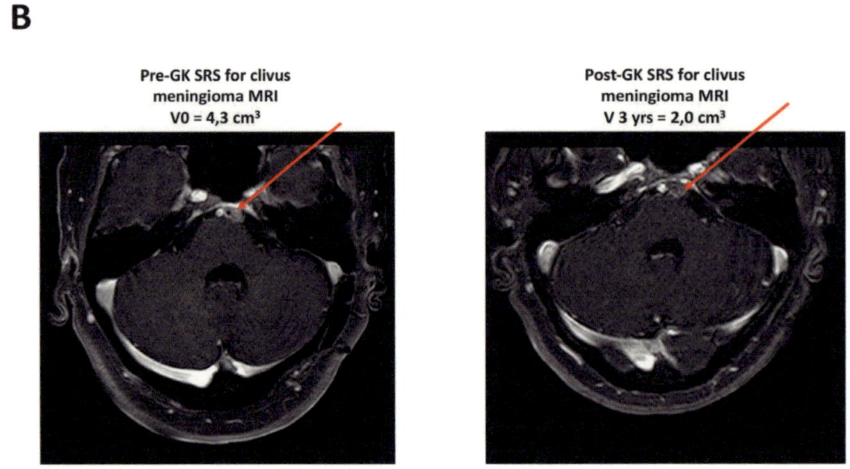

Figure 4.
A 45-year-old female with a clivus meningioma. She was treated in December 2012 with GK SRS 13.5 Gy, 50% isodose. At 3 years follow-up, there was a significant tumoral volume reduction (53.5% tumor reduction — Minor response according to response assessment in neuro-oncology [RANO] criteria) [77].

8.4 Study endpoints

Tumor volumes were calculated on T1 post-contrast MRI sequences using. Tumor stability (i.e., tumor control) was defined according to the RANO criteria [77].

8.5 Statistical analysis

Statistical analyses were performed with GraphPad Prism 9 and IBM SPSS statistics.

For all statistical tests, a p-value of <0.05 was considered as statistically significant. Change in meningioma volume at last brain MRI was compared to the pre-GKRS MRI before SRS.

9. Results

In our study, we collected 43 cases of IM treated with single-dose GK SRS. All the patients were hospitalized for 1 day for stereotactic neuroimage acquisition and then treated in an ambulatory setting. A total of 70% were skull base meningioma, and 30% were non-skull base meningioma. The prescription dose ranges between 12 and 15 Gy at an isodose of 35–60%, mean dose of 12.8 Gy, and a mean isodose of 48.3% (**Table 3**). Only one patient from the non-skull base IM presented transient edema as a complication of SRS (2.3%). Our results showed that there is a statistically significant tumor volume reduction in the skull base IM group (mean initial volume: 5.32 cm^3/last follow-up volume: 4.34 cm^3) as shown in **Figure 5A**. This tendency was not evident in the non-skull base group (mean initial volume: 5.78 cm^3/last follow-up volume: 5.36 cm^3). Also, at the volumetric follow-up, all the patients at least achieved a stable disease according to RANO, as shown in **Figure 5B**. The mean tumor volume change at 24 months post SRS was −10,6 and −23,9% for non-SB and SB meningiomas, respectively.

Factor		Total: 43
Sex (n, %)	**Male**	**6 (14%)**
	Female	**37 (86%)**
Age in years (mean ± SD, range)		54.7 ± 14.2 (30–85)
Initial tumor volume (n, %)	< 5 cm^3	25 (58%)
	5–10 cm^3	12 (28%)
	> 10 cm^3	6 (14%)
	Tumor volume in cm^3 (mean ± SD, range)	5.4 ± 4.7 (0.6–25.2)
Tumor localization	Skull base (n, %)	30 (70%)
	Tentorium (n)	8
	Cerebellopontine angle (n)	6
	Petroclival (n)	6
	Clivus (n)	3
	Sphenoidal (n)	3
	Cavernous sinus (n)	2
	Other skull base (n)	2
	Non-skull base (n, %)	13 (30%)
	Falx(n)	9
	Convexity (n)	2
	Parasagittal (n)	2
Prescription margin dose (Gy) (Mean ± SD, range)		12.8 ± 0.72 (12–15)
Isodose (%) (Mean ± SD, range)		48.3 ± 4.72 (35–60)

Table 3.
Demographics for the IM patients who underwent GK SRS. SD, standard deviation.

10. Discussion of our results

Our small series shows similar results to the literature (as shown in this review). To our knowledge, this is the first Chilean report of IM patients' outcomes with GK SRS. All the patients were managed in an ambulatory setting. In our series, there was a low incidence of SRS-related compilations. The long-term outcomes were satisfactory because all the samples achieved at least a stable disease stage. This means that the radiosurgical procedure could achieve tumor control as shown in **Figure 5B**.

Interestingly, the skull base group showed a statistically significant tumor volume reduction, as well as other reported series [37].

Of the collected cases, the most common IM treated with GK SRS was skull base IM. Among these, more than 50% were tentorial, cerebellopontine angle, and petroclival meningiomas. The posterior fossa tumors are located in a critical region considering the presence of the brainstem, and in close relation with cranial nerves and vertebrobasilar circulation. Moreover, IM surgery is associated with more complications which may explain why SRS is preferred for skull base compared to non-skull base IM.

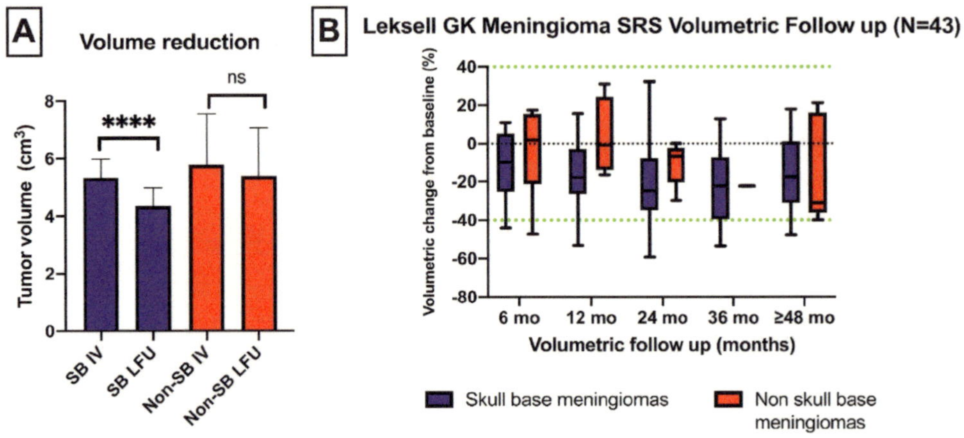

Figure 5.
A: Meningioma tumor volume changes before and after GK SRS (at last follow-up period). Separated by skull base and non-skull base meningiomas. Wilcoxon matched-pair signed rank test showed a statistically significant tumor volume reduction in skull base meningioma group after GK (p-value of p < 0,0001); but this result was not evident in the non-skull base group (p = 0.0764). Column graph with mean and SEM. B: Longitudinal follow-up of meningioma tumor volume subsequent to treatment with GK SRS, spanning a duration exceeding 48 months. Importantly, all participants demonstrated a status of at least stable disease, as determined by the RANO criteria. Grouped graph with box and whiskers type showing minimum and maximum data. IV, initial volume; LFU, last follow-up; SB, skull base.

From an economic perspective, several reports have revealed that SRS treatment is less expensive than microsurgery [78–80]. The Dutch study of Tan et al. demonstrated that initial treatment cost is about five times higher for microsurgery ($12,288 euros) compared to SRS ($1547 euros for LINAC radiosurgery and $2412 euros for GK radiosurgery) [79].

For this reason, our attention is directed toward SRS as an economically viable treatment option within the domain of public health and neurosurgery. By prioritizing SRS, we aim to adopt a therapeutic approach that not only proves effective in addressing health issues but also demonstrates cost-effectiveness on a larger scale and well-being of individuals.

There are several limitations of this study, first, it is a retrospective case series of a single-center experience. Also, there is a low consecutive follow-up of patients that diminished our sample size of collected cases.

11. Conclusion

In conclusion, primary SRS emerges as a safe and valuable therapeutic option for addressing small to medium-sized symptomatic intracranial meningiomas. It boasts a high degree of tumor control while maintaining low complication rates and ensuring favorable long-term functional outcomes. It is indicated in tumors classified as WHO grade I IM that cannot be resected without important morbidity and mortality, in patients that are poor surgical candidates or by patient preferences with delayed and low radiotoxicity. Also, SRS can be used as adjuvant therapy in gross total and subtotal resection as well as recurrent small IM. It is also useful but with lower control rates in WHO grade II or III residual operated tumors with more but reasonable morbidity. Permanent morbidity is low from 5.7%. There is an alternative hypofractionated SRS for large WHO grade I tumors or that are near organs at risk with good local control and low morbidity. SRS also has a place in difficult tumors, such as radiation-induced meningiomas, to achieve local control, especially in WHO grade I that progress after surgery or as primary in poor surgical candidates with acceptable toxicity.

Furthermore, as an ambulatory therapy from an epidemiological point of view, this approach can be used to treat selected IM patients, thereby reducing the waiting list. This is especially important in countries with less neurosurgical facilities achieving a safe and low toxicity technique.

Author details

Gustavo Zomosa[1,2*], Claudio Lühr[1], Francisco Bova[1], Lucas González-Johnson[2,3,4], Catalina Rojas-Solé[3], Lene Troncoso[3], Gonzalo Miranda[2] and José Lorenzoni[5]

1 Gamma Knife Center Chile, Santiago, Chile

2 Department of Neurology and Neurosurgery, Hospital Clínico Universidad de Chile, Santiago, Chile

3 Facultad de Medicina, Universidad de Chile, Santiago, Chile

4 Hospital Clínico Universidad de Chile, Santiago, Chile

5 Facultad de Medicina, Pontificia Universidad Católica de Chile, Santiago, Chile

*Address all correspondence to: gzomosar@hotmail.com

References

[1] Pikis S, Mantziaris G, Dumot C, Xu Z, Sheehan J. Stereotactic radiosurgery for intracranial meningiomas. Neurosurgery Clinics of North America. 2023;**34**(3):455-462. DOI: 10.1016/j.nec.2023.02.010

[2] Ostrom QT, Cioffi G, Waite K, Kruchko C, Barnholtz-Sloan JS. CBTRUS statistical report: Primary brain and other central nervous system tumors diagnosed in the United States in 2014-2018. Neuro-Oncology. 2021;**23**(Suppl. 3):iii1-iii105. DOI: 10.1093/neuonc/noab200

[3] Whittle IR, Smith C, Navoo P, Collie D. Meningiomas. Lancet London, England. 2004;**363**(9420):1535-1543. DOI: 10.1016/S0140-6736(04)16153-9

[4] Meling TR, Da Broi M, Scheie D, Helseth E. Meningiomas: skull base versus non-skull base. Neurosurgical Review. 2019;**42**(1):163-173. DOI: 10.1007/s10143-018-0976-7

[5] Magill ST, Young JS, Chae R, Aghi MK, Theodosopoulos PV, McDermott MW. Relationship between tumor location, size, and WHO grade in meningioma. Neurosurgical Focus. 2018;**44**(4):E4. DOI: 10.3171/2018.1.FOCUS17752

[6] Liang R-F et al. The potential risk factors for atypical and anaplastic meningiomas: Clinical series of 1,239 cases. International Journal of Clinical and Experimental Medicine. 2014;7(12):5696-5700

[7] Bos D et al. Prevalence, clinical management, and natural course of incidental findings on brain MR images: The population-based Rotterdam scan study. Radiology. 2016;**281**(2):507-515. DOI: 10.1148/radiol.2016160218

[8] Nakasu S, Nakasu Y. Natural history of meningiomas: Review with meta-analyses. Neurologia Medico-Chirurgica (Tokyo). 2020;**60**(3):109-120. DOI: 10.2176/nmc.ra.2019-0213

[9] Yano S, Kuratsu J, Kumamoto Brain Tumor Research Group. Indications for surgery in patients with asymptomatic meningiomas based on an extensive experience. Journal of Neurosurgery. 2006;**105**(4):538-543. DOI: 10.3171/jns.2006.105.4.538

[10] Ostrom QT, Gittleman H, Truitt G, Boscia A, Kruchko C, Barnholtz-Sloan JS. CBTRUS statistical report: Primary brain and other central nervous system tumors diagnosed in the United States in 2011-2015. Neuro-Oncology. 2018;**20**(suppl_4):iv1-iv86. DOI: 10.1093/neuonc/noy131

[11] Adekanmbi A et al. "Clinical management of supratentorial non-skull base meningiomas". Cancers. 2022;**14**(23):23. DOI : 10.3390/cancers14235887

[12] Flannery T, Poots J. Gamma knife radiosurgery for meningioma. Progress in Neurological Surgery. 2019;**34**:91-99. DOI: 10.1159/000493054

[13] Leksell L. The stereotaxic method and radiosurgery of the brain. Acta Chirurgica Scandinavica. 1951;**102**(4):316-319

[14] Kondziolka D, Shin SM, Brunswick A, Kim I, Silverman JS. The biology of radiosurgery and its clinical applications for brain tumors. Neuro-Oncology. 2015;**17**(1):29-44. DOI: 10.1093/neuonc/nou284

[15] Goldbrunner R et al. EANO guideline on the diagnosis and management

of meningiomas. Neuro-Oncology. 2021;**23**(11):1821-1834. DOI: 10.1093/neuonc/noab150

[16] Mathiesen T, Pettersson-Segerlind J, Kihlström L, Ulfarsson E. Meningiomas engaging major venous sinuses. World Neurosurgery. 2014;**81**(1):116-124. DOI: 10.1016/j.wneu.2013.01.095

[17] Haselsberger K et al. Staged gamma knife radiosurgery for large critically located benign meningiomas: Evaluation of a series comprising 20 patients. Journal of Neurology, Neurosurgery, and Psychiatry. 2009;**80**(10):1172-1175. DOI: 10.1136/jnnp.2008.156745

[18] Marchetti M et al. Stereotactic radiosurgery for intracranial noncavernous sinus benign meningioma: International stereotactic radiosurgery society systematic review, meta-analysis and practice guideline. Neurosurgery. 2020;**87**(5):879-890. DOI: 10.1093/neuros/nyaa169

[19] Sheehan J et al. An international multicenter matched cohort analysis of incidental meningioma progression during active surveillance or after stereotactic radiosurgery: The IMPASSE study. Neuro-Oncology. 2022;**24**(1):116-124. DOI: 10.1093/neuonc/noab132

[20] Kollová A, Liscák R, Novotný J, Vladyka V, Simonová G, Janousková L. Gamma knife surgery for benign meningioma. Journal of Neurosurgery. 2007;**107**(2):325-336. DOI: 10.3171/JNS-07/08/0325

[21] Kondziolka D, Lunsford LD, Flickinger JC. The application of stereotactic radiosurgery to disorders of the brain. Neurosurgery. 2008;**62**(Suppl. 2):707-719; discussion 719-720,. DOI: 10.1227/01.neu.0000316275.12962.0e

[22] Kondziolka D et al. Radiosurgery as definitive management of intracranial meningiomas. Neurosurgery. 2008;**62**(1):53-58; discussion 58-60,. DOI: 10.1227/01.NEU.0000311061.72626.0D

[23] Santacroce A et al. Long-term tumor control of benign intracranial meningiomas after radiosurgery in a series of 4565 patients. Neurosurgery. 2012;**70**(1):32. DOI: 10.1227/NEU.0b013e31822d408a

[24] Kondziolka D et al. Stereotactic radiosurgery for convexity meningiomas: Clinical article. Journal of Neurosurgery. 2009;**111**(3):458-463. DOI: 10.3171/2008.8.JNS17650

[25] Ding D, Xu Z, McNeill IT, Yen C-P, Sheehan JP. Radiosurgery for parasagittal and parafalcine meningiomas. Journal of Neurosurgery. 2013;**119**(4):871-877. DOI: 10.3171/2013.6.JNS13110

[26] Sheehan JP, Lee C-C, Xu Z, P rzybylowski CJ, Melmer PD, Schlesinger D. Edema following gamma knife radiosurgery for parasagittal and parafalcine meningiomas. Journal of Neurosurgery. 2015;**123**(5):1287-1293. DOI: 10.3171/2014.12.JNS142159

[27] Martínez Álvarez R. Radiocirugía en meningiomas de convexidad y parasagitales. In: Radiocirugía. Fundamentos, avances tecnológicos, indicaciones y resultados. 1 st ed. Spain: Grupo Arán; 2012. pp. 149-156

[28] Kreil W, Luggin J, Fuchs I, Weigl V, Eustacchio S, Papaefthymiou G. Long term experience of gamma knife radiosurgery for benign skull base meningiomas. Journal of Neurology, Neurosurgery, and Psychiatry. 2005;**76**(10):1425-1430. DOI: 10.1136/jnnp.2004.049213

[29] Flannery TJ et al. Long-term control of petroclival meningiomas through radiosurgery. Journal of Neurosurgery. 2010;**112**(5):957-964. DOI: 10.3171/2009.8.JNS09695

[30] Bin Alamer O et al. Stereotactic radiosurgery in the management of petroclival meningiomas: A systematic review and meta-analysis of treatment outcomes of primary and adjuvant radiosurgery. Journal of Neuro-Oncology. 2022;**157**(2):207-219. DOI: 10.1007/s11060-021-03934-0

[31] Lee C-C et al. Stereotactic radiosurgery for benign (World Health Organization grade I) cavernous sinus meningiomas-international stereotactic radiosurgery society (ISRS) practice guideline: A systematic review. Neurosurgery. 2018;**83**(6):1128-1142. DOI: 10.1093/neuros/nyy009

[32] Martinez-Perez R, Florez-Perdomo W, Freeman L, Ung TH, Youssef AS. Long-term disease control and treatment outcomes of stereotactic radiosurgery in cavernous sinus meningiomas. Journal of Neuro-Oncology. 2021;**152**(3):439-449. DOI: 10.1007/s11060-021-03732-8

[33] Cohen-Inbar O, Tata A, Moosa S, Lee C-C, Sheehan JP. Stereotactic radiosurgery in the treatment of parasellar meningiomas: Long-term volumetric evaluation. Journal of Neurosurgery. 2018;**128**(2):362-372. DOI: 10.3171/2016.11.JNS161402

[34] Xu D et al. Gamma knife surgery in the management of orbital tumors. Journal of Neurosurgery. 2010;**113**(Suppl.):34-38. DOI: 10.3171/2010.7.GKS10857

[35] Umekawa M, Shinya Y, Hasegawa H, Katano A, Saito N. Primary stereotactic radiosurgery provides favorable tumor control for intraventricular meningioma: A retrospective analysis. Journal of Clinical Medicine. 2023;**12**(3):1068. DOI: 10.3390/jcm12031068

[36] Starke RM, Williams BJ, Hiles C, Nguyen JH, Elsharkawy MY, Sheehan JP. Gamma knife surgery for skull base meningiomas. Journal of Neurosurgery. 2012;**116**(3):588-597. DOI: 10.3171/2011.11.JNS11530

[37] Vera E et al. A review of stereotactic radiosurgery practice in the management of skull base meningiomas. Journal of Neurological Surgery Part B: Skull Base. 2014;**75**(3):152-158. DOI: 10.1055/s-0033-1354747

[38] Nicolato A et al. Gamma knife radiosurgery in meningiomas of the posterior fossa. Experience with 62 treated lesions. Minimally Invasive Neurosurgery. 2001;**44**(4):211-217. DOI: 10.1055/s-2001-19934

[39] Patibandla MR, Lee C, Tata A, Addagada GC, Sheehan JP. Stereotactic radiosurgery for WHO grade I posterior fossa meningiomas: Long-term outcomes with volumetric evaluation. Journal of Neurosurgery. 2018;**129**(5):1249-1259. DOI: 10.3171/2017.6.JNS17993

[40] Nakao N, Ohkawa T, Miki J, Ogura M, Itakura T. Surgical treatment and outcome of skull base meningiomas with extracranial extensions. Clinical Neurology and Neurosurgery. 2010;**112**(1):40-46. DOI: 10.1016/j.clineuro.2009.10.003

[41] Corniola MV et al. Management of cavernous sinus meningiomas: Consensus statement on behalf of the EANS skull base section. Brain Spine. 2022;**2**:100864. DOI: 10.1016/j.bas.2022.100864

[42] Klinger DR, Flores BC, Lewis JJ, Barnett SL. The treatment of cavernous sinus meningiomas: Evolution of a modern approach. Neurosurgical Focus. 2013;**35**(6):E8. DOI: 10.3171/2013.9.FOCUS13345

[43] Sindou M, Wydh E, Jouanneau E, Nebbal M, Lieutaud T. Long-term follow-up of meningiomas of the cavernous sinus after surgical treatment alone. Journal of Neurosurgery. 2007;**107**(5):937-944. DOI: 10.3171/JNS-07/11/0937

[44] Lee JYK, Niranjan A, McInerney J, Kondziolka D, Flickinger JC, Lunsford LD. Stereotactic radiosurgery providing long-term tumor control of cavernous sinus meningiomas. Journal of Neurosurgery. 2002;**97**(1):65-72. DOI: 10.3171/jns.2002.97.1.0065

[45] Martínez Álvarez R. Radiocirugía en meningiomas de base de cráneo. In: Radiocirugía. Fundamentos, avances tecnológicos, indicaciones y resultados. 1 st. ed. Spain: Grupo Arán; 2012. pp. 137-147

[46] Zomosa R, Cruz S, Miranda G, Harbst H. Meningioma de la vaina del nervio óptico y tratamiento con radioterapia conformacional. Reporte de un caso clínico tratado con largo seguimiento. Revista Chilena de Neurocirugía. 2016;**42**:133-136

[47] Eddleman CS, Liu JK. Optic nerve sheath meningioma: Current diagnosis and treatment. Neurosurgical Focus. 2007;**23**(5):E4. DOI: 10.3171/FOC-07/11/E4

[48] Berman D, Miller NR. New concepts in the management of optic nerve sheath meningiomas. Annals of the Academy of Medicine, Singapore. 2006;**35**(3):168-174

[49] Turbin RE, Pokorny K. Diagnosis and treatment of orbital optic nerve sheath meningioma. Cancer Control. 2004;**11**(5):334-341. DOI: 10.1177/107327480401100508

[50] Kwon Y et al. Visual changes after gamma knife surgery for optic nerve tumors. Report of three cases. Journal of Neurosurgery. 2005;**102**(Suppl):143-146. DOI: 10.3171/jns.2005.102.s_supplement.0143

[51] Baumert BG et al. Early improvements in vision after fractionated stereotactic radiotherapy for primary optic nerve sheath meningioma. Radiotherapy and Oncology. 2004;**72**(2):169-174. DOI: 10.1016/j.radonc.2004.04.008

[52] Pereira BJA, de Almeida AN, Paiva WS, de Aguiar PHP, Teixeira MJ, Marie SKN. Natural history of intraventricular meningiomas: Systematic review. Neurosurgical Review. 2020;**43**(2):513-523. DOI: 10.1007/s10143-018-1019-0

[53] Lin M et al. Exoscopic resection of atrial intraventricular meningiomas using a navigation-assisted channel-based trans-sulcal approach: Case series and literature review. Journal of Clinical Neuroscience. 2020;**71**:58-65. DOI: 10.1016/j.jocn.2019.10.017

[54] Jamshidi AO, Beer-Furlan A, Hardesty DA, Ditzel Filho LFS, Prevedello LM, Prevedello DM. Management of large intraventricular meningiomas with minimally invasive port technique: A three-case series. Neurosurgical Review. 2021;**44**(4):2369-2377. DOI: 10.1007/s10143-020-01409-w

[55] Kim I-Y, Kondziolka D, Niranjan A, Flickinger JC, Lunsford LD. Gamma knife radiosurgery for intraventricular

meningiomas. Acta Neurochirurgica. 2009;**151**(5):447-452, 452. discussion. DOI: 10.1007/s00701-009-0273-x

[56] Daza-Ovalle A, Bin-Alamer O, Flickinger J, Niranjan A, Lunsford LD. Outcomes after gamma knife radiosurgery for intraventricular meningiomas. Journal of Neuro-Oncology. 2022;**160**(1):23-31. DOI: 10.1007/s11060-022-04091-8

[57] Milano MT et al. Radiation-induced edema after single-fraction or multifraction stereotactic radiosurgery for meningioma: A critical review. International Journal of Radiation Oncology, Biology, Physics. 2018;**101**(2):344-357. DOI: 10.1016/j.ijrobp.2018.03.026

[58] Novotný J, Kollová A, Liscák R. Prediction of intracranial edema after radiosurgery of meningiomas. Journal of Neurosurgery. 2006;**105**(Suppl):120-126. DOI: 10.3171/sup.2006.105.7.120

[59] Louis DN et al. The 2021 WHO classification of tumors of the central nervous system: A summary. Neuro-Oncology. 2021;**23**(8):1231-1251. DOI: 10.1093/neuonc/noab106

[60] Pasquier D, Rezvoy N. Atypical and malignant meningiomas. In: Belkacémi Y, Mirimanoff R-O, Ozsahin M, editors. Management of Rare Adult Tumours. Paris: Springer; 2010. pp. 19-27. DOI: 10.1007/978-2-287-92246-6_2

[61] Pasquier D et al. Atypical and malignant meningioma: Outcome and prognostic factors in 119 irradiated patients. A multicenter, retrospective study of the rare cancer network. International Journal of Radiation Oncology, Biology, Physics. 2008;**71**(5):1388-1393. DOI: 10.1016/j.ijrobp.2007.12.020

[62] Aghi MK et al. Long-term recurrence rates of atypical meningiomas after gross total resection with or without postoperative adjuvant radiation. Neurosurgery. 2009;**64**(1):56-60, 60. discussion. DOI: 10.1227/01.NEU.0000330399.55586.63

[63] Yang S-Y, Park C-K, Park S-H, Kim DG, Chung YS, Jung H-W. Atypical and anaplastic meningiomas: Prognostic implications of clinicopathological features. Journal of Neurology, Neurosurgery, and Psychiatry. 2008;**79**(5):574-580. DOI: 10.1136/jnnp.2007.121582

[64] Attia A et al. Patterns of failure after treatment of atypical meningioma with gamma knife radiosurgery. Journal of Neuro-Oncology. 2012;**108**(1):179-185. DOI: 10.1007/s11060-012-0828-1

[65] Valery CA et al. Grade II meningiomas and gamma knife radiosurgery: Analysis of success and failure to improve treatment paradigm. Journal of Neurosurgery. 2016;**125**(Suppl. 1):89-96. DOI: 10.3171/2016.7.GKS161521

[66] Helis CA et al. Stereotactic radiosurgery for atypical and anaplastic meningiomas. World Neurosurgery. 2020;**144**:e53-e61. DOI: 10.1016/j.wneu.2020.07.211

[67] Sethi RA et al. Dose-response relationships for meningioma radiosurgery. American Journal of Clinical Oncology. 2015;**38**(6):600-604. DOI: 10.1097/COC.0000000000000008

[68] Pollock BE, Stafford SL, Link MJ, Garces YI, Foote RL. Stereotactic radiosurgery of World Health Organization grade II and III intracranial meningiomas: Treatment results on the basis of a 22-year experience. Cancer. 2012;**118**(4):1048-1054. DOI: 10.1002/cncr.26362

[69] Williams BJ, Salvetti DJ, Starke RM, Yen CP, Sheehan JP. Stereotactic radiosurgery for WHO II and III meningiomas: Analysis of long-term clinical and radiographic outcomes. Journal of Radiosurgery & SBRT. 2013;**2**(3):183-191

[70] Lehrer EJ et al. A review of the role of stereotactic radiosurgery and immunotherapy in the management of primary central nervous system tumors. Biomedicine. 2022;**10**(11):2977. DOI: 10.3390/biomedicines10112977

[71] Huang J et al. The interim result of a phase I/II study of nivolumab with or without ipilimumab in combination with multi-fraction stereotactic radiosurgery for recurrent, high-grade, radiation-relapsed meningioma. Journal of Clinical Oncology. 2022;**40**(16_suppl):2068-2068. DOI: 10.1200/JCO.2022.40.16_suppl.2068

[72] Co JL et al. Meningioma screening with MRI in childhood leukemia survivors treated with cranial radiation. International Journal of Radiation Oncology, Biology, Physics. 2019;**104**(3):640-643. DOI: 10.1016/j.ijrobp.2019.02.057

[73] Cahan WG, Woodard HQ, Higinbotham NL, Stewart FW, Coley BL. Sarcoma arising in irradiated bone: Report of eleven cases. 1948. Cancer. 1998;**82**(1):8-34. DOI: 10.1002/(sici)1097-0142(19980101)82:1<8::aid-cncr3>3.0.co;2-w

[74] Bunevicius A et al. Stereotactic radiosurgery for treatment of radiation-induced meningiomas: A multiinstitutional study. Journal of Neurosurgery. 2021;**135**(3):862-870. DOI: 10.3171/2020.7.JNS202064

[75] Huo M et al. Efficacy of stereotactic radiosurgery for radiation-induced meningiomas. Journal of Neuro-Oncology. 2020;**148**(2):299-305. DOI: 10.1007/s11060-020-03515-7

[76] Pinzi V et al. Hypofractionated radiosurgery for large or in critical-site intracranial meningioma: Results of a phase 2 prospective study. International Journal of Radiation Oncology, Biology, Physics. 2023;**115**(1):153-163. DOI: 10.1016/j.ijrobp.2022.08.064

[77] Huang RY et al. Proposed response assessment and endpoints for meningioma clinical trials: Report from the response assessment in neuro-oncology working group. Neuro-Oncology. 2019;**21**(1):26-36. DOI: 10.1093/neuonc/noy137

[78] Wellis G, Nagel R, Vollmar C, Steiger H-J. Direct costs of microsurgical management of radiosurgically amenable intracranial pathology in Germany: An analysis of meningiomas, acoustic neuromas, metastases and arteriovenous malformations of less than 3 cm in diameter. Acta Neurochirurgica. 2003;**145**(4):249-255. DOI: 10.1007/s00701-003-0007-4

[79] Tan SS et al. A microcosting study of microsurgery, LINAC radiosurgery, and gamma knife radiosurgery in meningioma patients. Journal of Neuro-Oncology. 2011;**101**(2):237-245. DOI: 10.1007/s11060-010-0243-4

[80] Schmieder K, Engelhardt M, Wawrzyniak S, Börger S, Becker K, Zimolong A. The impact of microsurgery, stereotactic radiosurgery and radiotherapy in the treatment of meningiomas depending on different localizations. GMS Health Technology Assessment. 2010;**6**:Doc02. DOI: 10.3205/hta000080

Chapter 5

Molecular Alterations, Histopathology and Squash Cytology of Meningioma

Amit Kumar Chowhan and Mousmi Agrawal

Abstract

Meningioma originates from the arachnoid cap cells of duramater. It is a slow growing tumour of Central Nervous System. It is seen more commonly in females at around 66 years of age. The most common genetic abnormality is monosomy of chromosome 22. Since the inception of World Health Organisation (WHO), meningioma was graded based on histo-morphological appearance. At present, they are categorised into 3 grades. This chapter describes the molecular alterations, histopathological grading, histopathological subtypes and squash cytology of meningioma.

Keywords: grading, meningioma, molecular alterations, squash cytology, subtypes

1. Introduction

Meningioma is a slow growing tumour of Central Nervous System (CNS) arising from the meninges of brain and spinal cord. They comprise majority of the primary CNS tumours. The tumour is more commonly seen in females, compared to males [1]. Apart from gender, the increased incidence is also noted in first degree relatives and the tumour has association with various genetic syndromes such as neurofibromatosis type 2 (NF2), Von Hippel Lindau (VHL) disease, multiple endocrine neoplasia type 1 (MEN1), Li-Fraumeni syndrome, Cowden syndrome and Gorlin syndrome [2].

The World Health Organisation (WHO) has graded meningioma into three grades and 15 subtypes, with each subtype having its own histopathological characteristics and molecular association [1]. Meningothelial subtype is the most common (63%) followed by transitional meningioma (19%) [3]. The clinical presentation depends upon the size and site of tumour. Smaller tumours are usually asymptomatic and are diagnosed incidentally. However, larger tumours cause symptoms and neurological deficits. Majority of the meningiomas are grade 1 (benign) and have favourable prognosis. Grade 2 meningioma (atypical) have a higher chance of recurrence whereas grade 3 meningioma (anaplastic/malignant) have worst prognosis [1].

2. History

- The earliest written record of meningioma dates back to 1614, when Felix Plater from the University of Basel performed an autopsy on Sir Caspar Bonecurtius [4].
- In the sixteenth century, first surgery was performed for removal of meningioma. However, the first successful surgery was done in the year 1770 by Anoine Luis and removed meningioma from convexity (parasagittal) plane [5].
- In 1835, the first skull-based meningioma was removed successfully by Zanobi Pecchioli, Professor of Surgery at the University of Siena [6].
- William Macewen, a Scottish surgeon, was also known for performing successful removal of dural based meningioma [7].
- In 1922, Harvey Cushing used the term "meningioma" to describe group of tumours that can develop anywhere along the neuraxis (brain and spinal cord) of the body, but share many of the features in common [4].
- Based on cell structure, Charles Oberling segregated meningioma into several subtypes, and over the years, other different types of meningiomas were identified by many scientists. Later on, in 1979, the first WHO "blue book" *Histological Typing of Tumours of the Central Nervous System* was released, which classified meningioma into seven subtypes, which got upgraded in its further editions 1993, 2000, 2007 and 2016. The latest fifth edition of "*WHO Classification of Tumours of the Central Nervous System (CNS)*" blue book, was published in 2021 and has graded meningioma into 3 different grades and described 15 histopathological subtypes of meningioma [8]. Each WHO "blue book" included revisions that reflected changes in concepts, knowledge, updates and represented an improvement over its previous editions.

3. Epidemiology

Meningiomas comprise 37.6% of primary CNS tumours. Meningiomas are more common with increasing age, 66 years being the median age of diagnosis. It is more commonly seen in females, compared to males, with female: male ratio of 2.3:1 [1].

Incidence rate ranges from 0.16/100,000 for patients aged 0 to 19 to 18.69/100,000 for those over 40 years. It has been observed that children present more frequently with high grade meningioma and have poor prognosis [9]. Typically, 2–3% of individuals have meningioma identified incidentally during autopsy [10].

According to WHO grading system of meningioma, 80–82% are grade 1, 17–18% comprise grade 2 and 1.7% forms grade 3 [1]. The recurrence rate of meningioma increases 2% every year, that is, at 10 years, the chances of recurrence increase by 20% [11]. According to the literature, higher-grade meningiomas have high recurrence rates. The recurrence rate in grade 3 meningiomas ranges approximately from 50 to 94%. In contrast, the recurrence rate in grades 1 and 2 meningioma is 7 to 25% and 29 to 52%, respectively [12].

4. Sites

4.1 CNS sites

Meningiomas most commonly arise in the cerebral convexities (parasagittal/ falx cerebri/venous sinuses). Other sites include olfactory grooves, sphenoid ridges, parasellar/suprasellar regions, optic nerve sheath, petrous ridges, tentorium and posterior fossa. Very rarely, they are found in intraventricular and epidural sites [13].

Few subtypes of meningioma have predilection for specific locations: [12, 14, 15].

- Meningothelial meningioma–midline or paramedian skull base
- Psammomatous meningioma–thoracic spine
- Chordoid meningioma–supratentorial
- Clear cell meningioma–cerebellopontine angle and spine especially cauda equina
- Papillary meningioma–supratentorial
- Rhabdoid meningioma–supratentorial, infratentorial or spinal
- Anaplastic meningioma–Cerebral or spinal meninges, cerebral ventricle

4.2 Ectopic sites

The most common ectopic site is head and neck region which includes scalp skin, intraosseous, orbit, paranasal sinuses, temporal bone and ear [16]. Very rarely, few cases have also been reported in lungs, salivary glands and mediastinum [17–19].

5. Pathophysiology

5.1 Pathogenesis

The origin of meningioma is from arachnoid cap cells of the duramater or choroid plexus. The most common genetic abnormality seen in majority of the meningioma is monosomy of chromosome 22 with more than 50% of tumours show allelic loss in 22q12.2, the region encoding the neurofibromatosis 2 (NF2) gene, also known as merlin gene [1]. On the contrary, paediatric meningiomas do not demonstrate NF2 mutations, instead they predominantly have YAP1 alterations, further leading to activation of the Hippo pathway [20].

A study of genomic sequencing was carried on sporadic meningioma and it revealed two subsets of mutations. The first subset had NF2 mutations and loss of chromosome 22. The second subset lacked NF2 mutation, but however manifested recurrent oncogenic mutations in AKT1 and PIK3CA. In addition, alterations in TRAF7, KLF4 and SMO were also observed [13, 21].

5.2 Diagnostic molecular pathology

The subtypes of meningioma are closely correlated with genetic changes (e.g. in AKT1, SMO, and PIK3CA), although these changes do not define them. DNA sequencing can be used to determine the status of the majority of genetic modifications that are directly relevant to subtyping and grading, including the TERT promoter, SMARCE1, KLF4 and TRAF7, and other abnormalities. The most malignant-appearing and proliferative sites should be the focus of tissue selection for DNA extraction because TERT mutations can develop throughout progression of disease. In situ hybridization can be used to detect homozygous deletion of CDKN2A and/or CDKN2B, or it can be computed using a variety of high-throughput sequencing or hybridization assays. However, it carries a limitation, as FISH probes are large, this method occasionally misses minor deletions. High-resolution copy-number plots may occasionally be used to infer rare events such as TERT activation by gene fusion or gene fusions involving YAP1, although RNA sequencing or in situ hybridization are often required for their confirmation. Because BAP1 and PBRM1 are susceptible to both mutation and deletion, DNA sequencing and independent copy-number analysis are required to analyse such mutations. Apart from DNA based methods, various immunohistochemical (IHC) stains can be used to detect genetic alterations such as SMARCE1 loss in clear cell meningioma and BAP1 loss in rhabdoid meningioma [14, 22]. Various diagnostic modalities used to assess genetic mutations in meningioma are summarised in **Table 1**.

5.3 Subtypes of meningioma and genetic alterations

It has been observed that certain types of meningioma have specific genetic alterations (summarised in **Table 2**).

5.4 Tumour location and mutation spectrum

Certain mutations have strong correlation with tumour site. While skull base meningiomas have mutations in AKT1, TRAF7, SMO, and/or PIK3CA, the convexity meningiomas and the majority of spinal meningiomas frequently have a 22q deletion and/or NF2 mutations [13]. Meningiomas harbouring 22q alterations (e.g. NF2, SMARCB1) originate from neural crest derived meninges and includes convexity, falx, tentorium and spinal cord. Whereas, the meningiomas driven by hedgehog signalling pathway, PI3K signalling, TRAF7, KLF4 and POLR2A mutations, arise from the mesoderm derived meninges of midline/paramedian anterior, central and ventral skull base [24].

Diagnostic methods	Genetic mutations
Immunohistochemistry	SMARCE1 loss in clear cell meningioma and BAP1 loss in rhabdoid meningioma
DNA sequencing	TERT promoter, SMARCE1, KLF4 and TRAF7
In situ hybridization	homozygous deletion of CDKN2A and/or CDKN2B
Copy-number plots	TERT activation, YAP1 gene fusions
DNA sequencing and copy-number analysis	BAP1 and PBRM1

Table 1.
List of methods for diagnosing genetic mutations in meningioma [14, 22].

Subtypes of meningioma	Genetic alterations
Meningothelial meningioma	AKT1, TRAF7, SMO, and/or PIK3CA mutations [13, 23]
Fibrous, transitional and psammomatous meningioma	22q deletion and NF2 allele mutation [14, 24]
Secretory meningioma	KLF4/TRAF7 mutation [22]
Angiomatous, microcystic, and metaplastic meningioma	Gain of chromosome 5 [25]
Chordoid meningioma	Deletion of chromosome 2p [26]
Clear cell meningioma	Both germline and somatic SMARCE1 mutations [27]
Papillary and rhabdoid meningioma	PBRM1 and BAP1 mutation or deletion [14]
Anaplastic meningioma	Mainly NF2 inactivation by mutation or chromosome 22q loss [14]; other alterations includes TERT promoter mutation, homozygous deletion of CDKN2A and/or CDKN2B and loss of H3 p.K28me3 (K27me3) [28–30]

Table 2.
Genetic alterations observed in meningioma subtypes.

6. Aetiology

Certain risk factors are attributed for increasing and decreasing the size of tumour.

6.1 Risk factors leading to increase in size of tumour

i. Ionising radiation, either low dose or high dose, especially for chordoid and anaplastic meningiomas [31, 32]

ii. Hormone replacement therapy or oral contraceptives [33]

iii. Excess body fat (obesity) and alcohol [34]

iv. History of prior surgery, male gender, especially in non-skull based atypical meningioma [35]

v. Long term progestin therapy responsible for enrichment of PIK3CA mutations [36]

vi. Mutations in SMARCB1 and SMARCE1 predispose to multiple meningiomas [37]

vii. Breast cancer [2]

6.2 Factors leading to decrease in size of tumour

i. Breastfeeding for ≥6 months [2, 38]

ii. Allergic diseases such as asthma and eczema [39]

7. Clinical presentation

Majority of the meningiomas are diagnosed in females at around 60–65 years, however, there are some exceptions [1]. Chordoid meningioma can be seen in adults, with average age at diagnosis being 45 years [14]. Clear cell meningioma is mostly seen in children and younger population, median age at diagnosis being 24 years [15]. Papillary meningioma is seen in both children and adults [14].

Meningiomas are slow growing tumours and can cause a variety of neurological impairments, depending upon the tumour's location. Small tumours are usually asymptomatic and diagnosed incidentally during autopsy. Larger tumours cause compression of nearby structures and produce clinical signs and symptoms. Typical symptoms of meningiomas include headaches, weakness, and convulsions [40].

However, there are few specific symptoms seen in meningioma attributed to their certain locations. Meningioma that cover the cerebrum, sphenoid bone, supra orbital bone or cavernous sinus may produce seizures. Tumours extending into the parasagittal region cause progressive spastic weakness/paralysis in the contralateral limbs and urinary incontinence [41]. Tumours of the Sylvian aqueduct or ventricles can induce a wide range of motor, sensory, aphasic and seizure symptoms. Further, rise in intracranial pressure and hydrocephalus can also occur [42]. Spinal meningiomas cause pain, radiculopathy and local site tenderness. Symptoms include decreased muscle tone, weakness, muscle fasciculations and hyporeflexia [43].

7.1 Metastasis

Anaplastic (malignant) meningiomas are aggressive in nature and have a higher chance to metastasize, although the incidence of meningioma metastasis is very rare (around 0.18%). Ideally, brain tumours do not metastasize to distant sites because of the protective blood brain barrier (BBB), but exceptionally anaplastic meningiomas can. The reason being, these tumours are located towards the blood side of BBB and they are directly connected to the blood vessels. Hence, the malignant cells escape into the blood stream and frequently metastasize into lungs [44]. Similarly, papillary meningioma display papillary growth architecture having propensity for brain invasion and producing dissemination and metastasis, primarily to the lung [14]. Apart from lungs, very rarely other metastatic sites are pleura, bones, liver, lymph node and kidney [10].

8. Diagnosis of meningioma

WHO CNS fifth edition has laid down certain "*essential and desirable diagnostic criteria*" for the diagnosis of meningioma: [14, 22].

8.1 Essential criteria

It includes classic histopathological features matching at least one of the meningioma subtypes *OR* suggestive histopathological features combined with biallelic inactivation of NF2 or other classic drivers of conventional meningioma (TRAF7, AKT1, KLF4, SMO, PIK3CA), clear cell meningioma (SMARCE1), or rhabdoid meningioma (BAP1) *OR s*uggestive of histopathological features combined with one of the defined DNA methylation classes of meningioma.

8.2 Desirable criteria

It includes tumour localised to meninges; EMA and SSTR2A positivity on immunohistochemistry; classic copy-number alterations of NF2-mutant meningioma, such as monosomy 22/22q in lower-grade meningiomas, with additional losses of 1p, 6, 10q, 14q, and/or 18 in higher-grade meningiomas.

9. ICD coding for meningioma

- ICD-O coding: 9530/0 Meningioma [14]
- ICD-11 coding: 2A01.0Z Meningiomas, unspecified

10. Evolution of grading system in meningioma

10.1 WHO CNS first edition (1979)

This edition included following categories of meningioma: meningotheliomatous (syncytial), fibrous, transitional, psammomatous, angiomatous, hemangioblastic, hemangiopericytoma, papillary and anaplastic meningioma [45, 46]. Strict criteria for WHO grade I, II and III were however not specified, but it suggested that tumours should be designated as grade II when following features are present: increased cellularity, frequent mitotic activity, high nucleus: cytoplasmic ratio, prominent nucleoli, patternless or sheet like growth and foci of necrosis (either spontaneous or geographic). Grade III meningiomas are anaplastic (malignant) in nature and should have features of malignancy in excess to that observed in grade II tumours [47].

10.2 WHO CNS second edition (1993)

In this edition, more new variants were added: microcystic, secretory, clear cell, chordoid, lymphoplasmacytic and metaplastic meningioma. Atypical meningioma was introduced as a category, but was not clearly defined. Further, Hemangioblastic category got deleted. Hemangiopericytoma was moved to "Mesenchymal, Non-Meningothelial Tumours" category [46]. Meningiomas were graded into three grades: I, II and III. Meningiomas categorised under grade I had low proliferative activity, distinct in nature and can be cured by surgical resection without any chance of recurrence. Grade II meningiomas had features similar as described in previous edition. Grade III meningiomas constitute anaplastic variant. These tumours are either anaplastic from the beginning or develop as a result of transition from grade I or II meningiomas and carry the highest tendency to metastasize [45].

10.3 WHO CNS third edition (2000)

A new variant rhabdoid meningioma was added and was categorised into grade III [48]. Further, the boundaries between benign and atypical meningioma and between atypical and malignant meningioma were not well delineated in the 1993 WHO classification. To address this issue, the 2000 WHO classification, recommended more objective criteria, which was largely based on a series of research from Mayo Clinic [49, 50].

Meningiomas having a low probability of recurrence and/or aggressive growth were included in WHO grade I. It included meningothelial meningioma, fibrous/fibroblastic meningioma, transitional (mixed), psammomatous meningioma, angiomatous meningioma, microcystic meningioma, secretory meningioma, lymphoplasmacyte-rich meningioma, and metaplastic meningioma. Meningiomas with a higher risk of recurrence and/or aggressive growth were classified by the WHO as grades II and III. Atypical meningioma, intracranial clear cell meningioma, and chordoid meningioma were all classified as WHO grade II. Rhabdoid meningioma, papillary meningioma, and anaplastic (malignant) meningioma were classified as WHO grade III. Further, it was recommended, that any subtype or grade of meningioma having high proliferative index and/or brain invasion should be additionally reported [48].

Indicators of tumour proliferation, like MIB-1 labelling index, are helpful in determining the likelihood of meningioma recurrence. Cut-off levels of MIB-1 labelling index distinguishing benign from atypical meningiomas and atypical from malignant meningiomas were not recommended, nonetheless, due to inter-institutional and inter-observer heterogeneity. However, high proliferation indices do offer independent predictive data of tumour recurrence. Therefore, it was advised that if the labelling indices were significantly higher than predicted, a term *"with high proliferative activity"* should be included to the diagnoses of benign or atypical meningioma [48].

Similarly, it has been demonstrated that grade 1 meningioma have an increased recurrence risk similar to an atypical meningioma, if there is presence of brain invasion [49, 50]. Additionally, the development of a malignant course cannot be necessarily predicted by the presence of brain invasion in an atypical meningioma. Hence, in the third edition, it was suggested that if brain invasion was present, a word *"with brain invasion"* should be included to the diagnosis of benign or atypical meningiomas. This will alert the clinician to a higher likelihood of recurrence, particularly in the case of a histologically benign (grade 1) meningioma [48].

10.4 WHO CNS fourth edition (2007)

There were no major changes. The only notable change to the WHO grading system in 2007 was the addition of brain invasion as a criteria for atypical meningioma, whereas in WHO third edition (2000) it was suggested as an additional finding to be included in reporting, if present [46, 51].

10.5 Updated WHO CNS fourth edition (2016)

The 2007 edition was further updated in 2016, however no substantial changes were observed in meningioma [46].

10.6 WHO CNS fifth edition (2021)

This edition introduces the major changes incorporating the molecular diagnostics in CNS tumour classification. Roman numerals (I, II, and III) were used to indicate the CNS WHO tumour grades in the past. But the latest fifth edition has recommended the use of Arabic numerals 1, 2, and 3 in the grading system. This change was to bring CNS tumour grades in line with other organ systems [22].

In WHO CNS fifth edition, meningioma is recognised as a single type, having further 15 subtypes reflecting its wide morphological variety. It is currently stressed that the criteria defining atypical or anaplastic (grade 2 or 3) meningioma should be implemented regardless of the underlying subtype. Whereas, chordoid and clear cell meningiomas have been solely placed in CNS WHO grade 2 as they are more likely to recur. Similarly, rhabdoid and papillary morphology are categorised into CNS WHO grade 3 [22].

Following is the WHO CNS 5 grading system for meningioma: [12, 14, 22].

a. *CNS WHO grade 1*: Tumours have low mitotic activity (< 4/10 high power field); brain invasion absent; < 3/5 atypical features (tumour necrosis, increased cellularity, small tumour cells with high nucleus: cytoplasmic ratio, sheet like growth and prominent large nucleoli).

b. *CNS WHO grade 2*: This includes intermediate mitotic count (4–19/10 high power field); presence of brain invasion; chordoid or clear cell histopathological subtype; at least presence of 3/5 atypical features (increased tumour cellularity, small tumour cells with high nucleus: cytoplasmic ratio, nucleoli prominence, sheet like or uninterrupted growth pattern, presence of spontaneous necrosis).

c. *CNS WHO grade 3*: Includes high mitotic activity (≥20/10 high power field); anaplastic histopathological features (sarcoma/carcinoma/melanoma–like morphology), TERT promoter mutation; homozygous deletion of CDKN2A and/or CDKN2B genes.

11. Errors in grading due to treatment related effects

Few hospitals perform preoperative embolization of meningioma to reduce intraoperative bleeding and the pathologist might not be informed regarding embolization procedure. The histological alterations caused by embolization, such as macro nucleoli, necrosis and compensatory proliferation with more mitotic figures, may result in the tumour being over graded. Over grading can be prevented through communication between the neurosurgeon and neuropathologist regarding the use of embolization. Similarly, acknowledging the patient's prior radiation therapy would help to allay features of necrosis or cellular atypia [52].

12. Macroscopic appearance

On gross appearance, majority of the meningiomas are well circumscribed, globular, solid masses attached to the underlying duramater. These tumours are firm to rubbery in consistency. Some meningiomas are lobulated or have bilobed appearance and grow in a flat en plaque like pattern along the dura of sphenoid bone. Few subtypes of meningioma have characteristic morphology which provides a clue in their diagnosis. Psammomatous meningiomas of the spinal region have gritty texture because of presence of psammoma bodies (calcified spherules). Fibrous meningioma has a smooth surface [14]. Chordoid meningioma have a soft, gelatinous, cystic consistency with a smooth contour and has translucent areas on cut surface. Atypical meningiomas are seen invading the adjacent brain parenchyma [35].

Majority of grade 1 meningiomas compress and displace the adjacent brain, but are neither adherent nor invasive, and thus can be easily removed. However, higher-grade meningiomas are widely adherent and invasive to the adjacent brain tissue and show necrotic changes. Sometimes, these tumours are able to infiltrate the dural sinuses as well. Parasagittal meningiomas have the ability to partially or totally block the superior sagittal sinus. Rarely, meningiomas can penetrate the skull bone and produce reactive hyperostosis of the skull vault. Cerebral arteries and/or cranial nerves may be attached to or encased by meningiomas, but are usually not infiltrated [12, 14].

13. Histopathological subtypes of meningioma

13.1 Meningothelial meningioma

This is the most common subtype of meningioma. The tumour cells resemble the morphology of arachnoid cap cells. The cells are arranged in syncytia like lobules separated by thin collagenous septae (**Figure 1a**). The cells are monomorphic, with

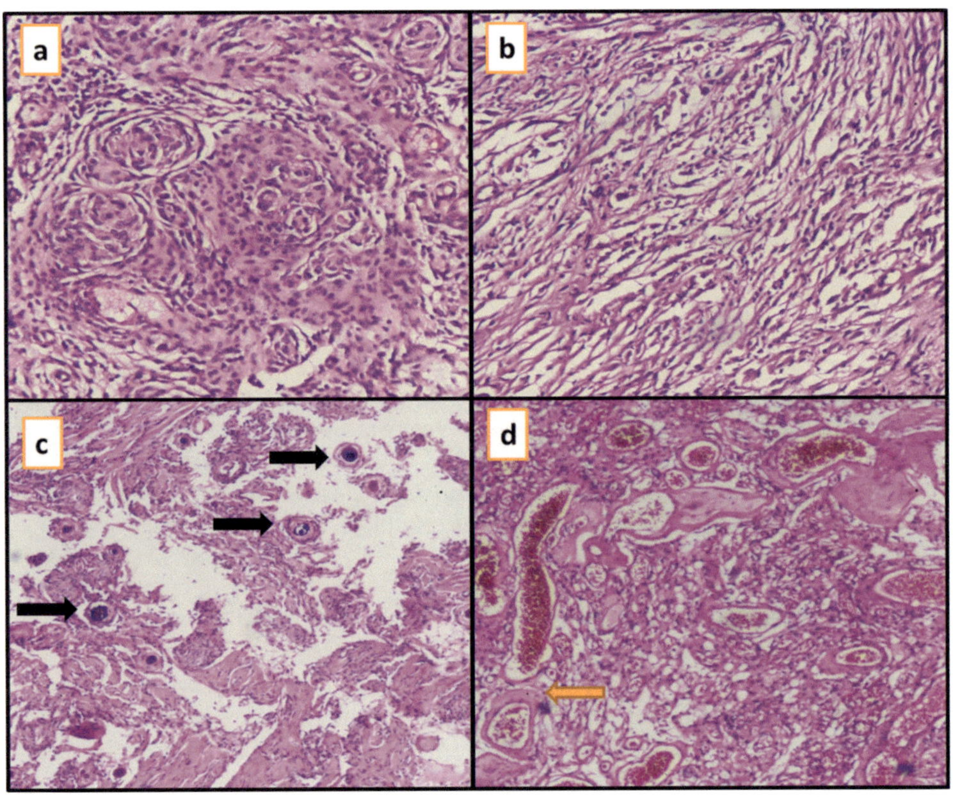

Figure 1.
Photomicrographs of (a) meningothelial meningioma having cells arranged in syncytia like lobules separated by thin collagenous septae (microscopic filed with 100X in haematoxylin and eosin stain); (b) fibrous meningioma characterised by spindle cells arranged in parallel and interlacing bundles (microscopic filed with 100X in haematoxylin and eosin stain); (c) Psammomatous meningioma displaying calcified psammoma bodies (black arrow, microscopic filed with 40X in haematoxylin and eosin stain); and (d) angiomatous meningioma having hyalinised thick walled blood vessels (orange arrow, microscopic filed with 40X in haematoxylin and eosin stain).

few cells having nuclear haloes, pseudo inclusions and eosinophilic cytoplasm. Very rarely, psammoma bodies and meningothelial whorls are noted [12, 14].

13.2 Fibrous meningioma

This subtype is characterised by spindle cells arranged in parallel, storiform, or interlacing bundles in a collagen-rich matrix (**Figure 1b**). The fascicles formed by tumour cells contain variable amounts of intercellular collagen [14, 24].

13.3 Transitional meningioma

This subtype has features of both meningothelial and fibrous patterns, as well as some transitional characteristics. There are places that have both lobular and fascicular architecture, with some of these areas being in between the two patterns (thus the term "transitional"). This subtype frequently exhibits whorls and psammoma bodies [12, 14].

13.4 Psammomatous meningioma

Psammoma bodies predominate over the tumour cells in this subtype. (**Figure 1c**). Sometimes, these psammoma bodies overlap each other and combine to form enormous, calcified masses. Although actual meningioma cells can be scarce and difficult to identify, immunohistochemistry markers for EMA or SSTR2A can highlight them. The non-calcified foci resemble the morphology of fibrous or transitional subtype [12, 14].

13.5 Angiomatous meningioma

This subtype is characterised by predominance of small blood vessels, which can be thick or thin walled and are variably hyalinised (**Figure 1d**). The actual meningioma tumour cells may be difficult to locate between these vessels. Additionally, microcytic or metaplastic areas can also be present, however the tumour cells of these regions show degenerative changes and nuclear atypia. Adjacent brain tissue shows oedematous changes [12, 14].

13.6 Microcystic meningioma

On histology, the microcystic subtype of meningioma comprises microcysts made of cells with thin, elongated processes that give the tissue a cobweb-like appearance (**Figure 2a**). The cysts may coalesce together and form large macrocyst. Degenerative nuclear atypia can also be observed in microcystic meningioma, just like in angiomatous meningioma, which raises the suspicion of a higher-grade tumour, however, this variant is benign in nature. Associated cerebral edema can be noticed [12, 14]. On immunohistochemistry, these microcystic areas are diffusely and weakly positive for carbonic anhydrase IX (hypoxic marker) [53].

13.7 Secretory meningioma

This subtype is characterised by gland like epithelial pattern, the lumen of which contains PAS positive eosinophilic secretions which resemble psammoma bodies, hence termed as pseudo psammoma bodies (**Figure 2b**). These secretions are positive

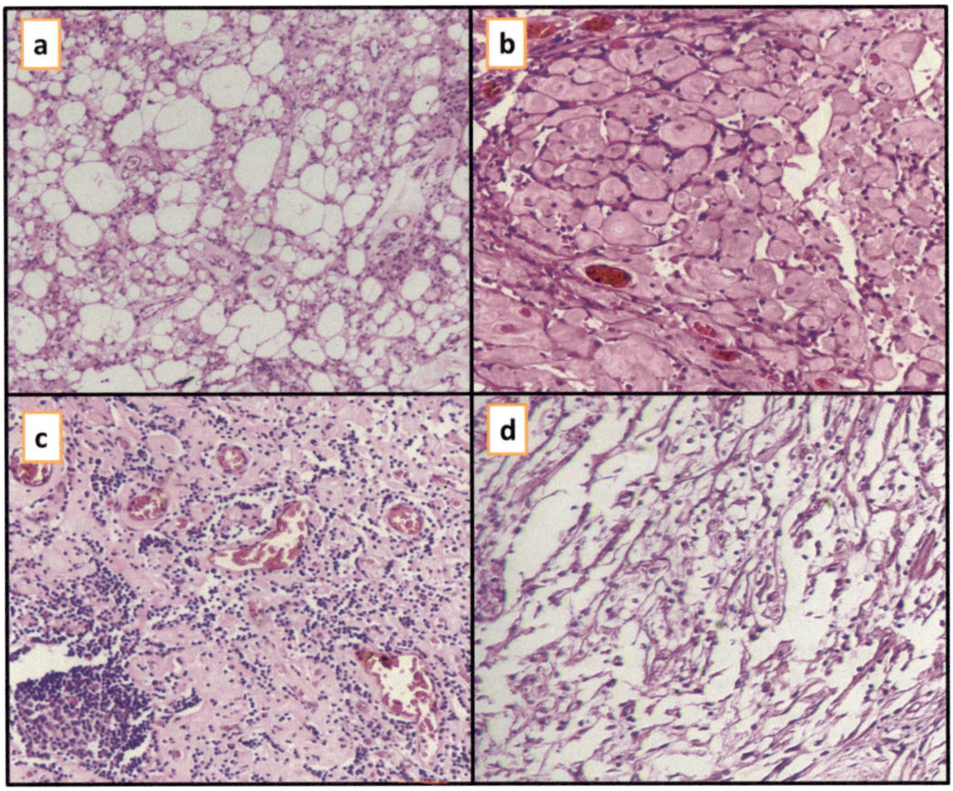

Figure 2.
Photomicrographs of (a) microcystic meningioma having microcysts with cobweb like appearance (microscopic filed with 40X in haematoxylin and eosin stain); (b) secretory meningioma characterised by gland like epithelial pattern with lumen containing eosinophilic secretions (microscopic filed with 100X in haematoxylin and eosin stain); (c) Lymphoplasmacyte-rich meningioma displaying dense collection of lymphocytes (microscopic filed with 100X in haematoxylin and eosin stain); and (d) clear cell meningioma having large polygonal clear cells with clear cytoplasm and presence of interstitial collagen (microscopic filed with 100X in haematoxylin and eosin stain).

for carcino embryonic antigen (CEA). Therefore, elevated CEA levels is observed in these patients, the levels fall down by resection and again rises up by recurrence of tumour. Peritumoral oedema is present. KLF4 and TRAF7 mutations are seen. The surrounding tumour cells are also positive for CEA and keratin [54].

13.8 Lymphoplasmacyte-rich meningioma

This subtype is very rare, seen in less than 1% cases. On histopathology, the tumour is characterised by presence of extensive chronic inflammatory cells, predominantly macrophages and very few plasma cells (**Figure 2c**). Meningothelial component is generally scant [55].

13.9 Metaplastic meningioma

This variant has presence of mesenchymal components which can be present singly or in combinations and it includes bone, cartilage, fat, myxoid or xanthomatous changes. However, this does not constitute true metaplasia and do not carry any clinical significance [12, 14].

13.10 Atypical meningioma

Atypical meningioma is categorised into CNS WHO grade 2. It is an intermediate grade meningioma. This subtype is characterised by brain invasion, which is described as irregular, tongue shaped protrusion of tumour cells into the brain parenchyma without intervening leptomeninges. Infiltration of tumour cells into the perivascular Virchow-Robin spaces does not come under brain invasion as piamater is not breached. Sometimes, it is difficult to locate brain parenchyma in between the tumour cells, in such cases immunohistochemistry marker GFAP is useful for highlighting intervening glial tissue [12, 14]. Studies say that these tumours have higher chances of recurrence despite total resection and show bony involvement [56, 57]. Interestingly, it should be noted that mere presence of bone involvement is not considered as a criteria for atypical meningioma.

13.11 Chordoid meningioma

This is a rare subtype accounting for 0.5–1% of intracranial meningiomas. The tumour has equal preponderance for both males and females [58]. The tumour is named "chordoid" because it resembles "chordoma" on histopathology, and is characterised by small epitheloid to spindled shaped tumour cells arranged in cords and trabeculae having foamy vacuolated cytoplasm embedded in a mucin rich matrix. Interspersed chronic inflammatory cells are also present [14, 59]. On immunohistochemistry, the tumour cells are positive for EMA, podoplanin and patchy cytokeratin whereas negative for S100, brachyury and GFAP [58]. Immunoreactivity with NHERF1 has also been reported [60]. Rarely these patients have associated comorbid haematological disorders like Castleman disease and anaemia [61].

Chordoid meningiomas have been designated as CNS WHO grade 2 because these tumours have high chance of recurrence. The increased recurrence risk is due to high proliferative activity and atypical histopathological features [58].

13.12 Clear cell meningioma

It is a rare variant and accounts for 0.2–0.8% of all meningiomas. This subtype has round to polygonal cells with clear, glycogen-rich cytoplasm and abundant perivascular and interstitial collagen (**Figure 2d**). The clear cells are arranged in pattern-less or sheet like architecture [14]. The cytoplasmic glycogen is PAS-positive and diastase-sensitive. Occasionally, perivascular and interstitial collagen combines to form large acellular eosinophilic collagen areas. Whorls and psammoma bodies are absent. Mitotic activity is not prominent [15]. On immunohistochemistry, the tumour cells are positive for EMA, PR and Vimentin. Characteristic loss of nuclear expression with SMARCE1 is noted [22]. Clear cell meningiomas are classified as CNS WHO grade 2 because of their association with more aggressive behaviour, recurrence and cerebrospinal fluid seeding [14]. Clear cell meningioma should be distinguished from metastatic clear cell renal cell carcinoma, the latter is strongly positive for keratin, EMA and negative for S100 protein [45].

13.13 Anaplastic (malignant) meningioma

Anaplastic meningioma is rare and comprises 1–3% of all meningiomas. It is designated under CNS WHO grade 3 category and has an aggressive malignant morphology. The tumours can invade brain parenchyma and show extensive necrosis (**Figure 3**). These tumours can be primary (arise de novo) or secondary (progress from grade 1 or 2 meningioma). Most of the time, due to higher grade morphology, meningothelial origin is difficult to identify, thus it can be confirmed by immunohistochemistry and/or genetic testing. On immunohistochemistry, the cells are positive for EMA, SSTR2A, focal CK AE1/AE3 and STAT6. Genetically, these tumours show TERT promoter mutation and homozygous deletion of CDKN2A and/or CDKN2B genes, which can by identified by molecular testing [14, 22].

The differentials of anaplastic meningioma include metastatic carcinoma, melanoma of meninges, sarcoma and solitary fibrous tumour (SFT). Immunohistochemistry plays a major role in distinguishing them. Metastatic carcinoma is strongly and diffusely positive with CK AE1/AE3. Meningeal melanoma will show brown coloured melanin pigment, which can be confirmed with melanin bleach and Fontana-Masson special stain. Further melanoma will be positive for HMB45, Melan A and negative for EMA.

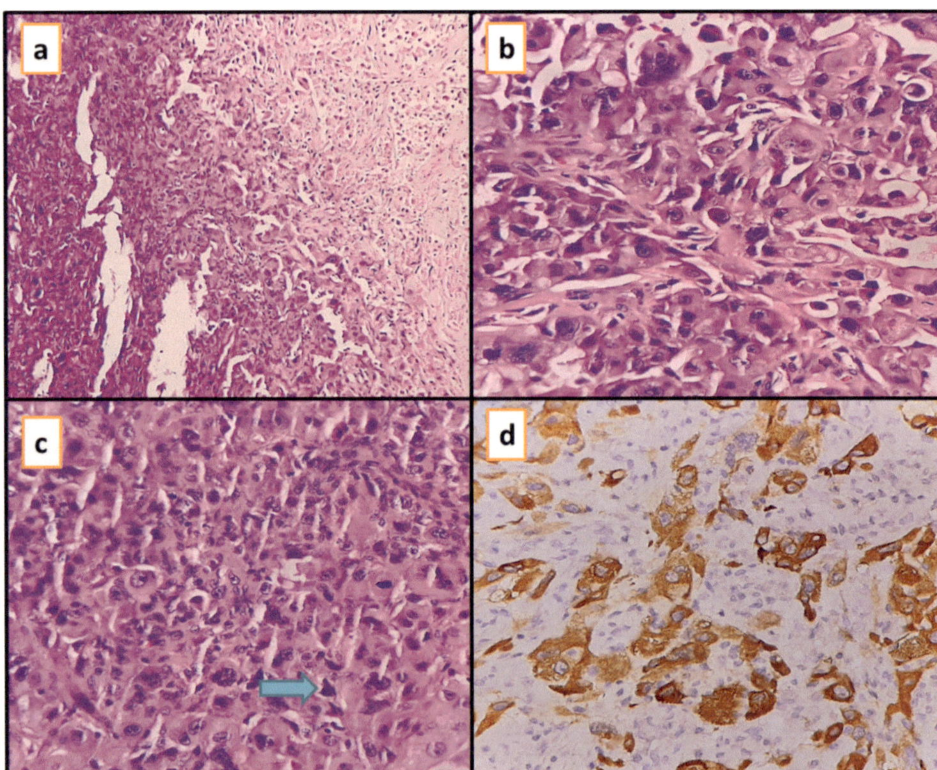

Figure 3.
Photomicrographs from a case of anaplastic meningioma (a) tumour necrosis (microscopic filed with 100X in haematoxylin and eosin stain), (b) malignant cells with large prominent nucleoli and bizzare morphology (microscopic filed with 400X in haematoxylin and eosin stain), (c) atypical tripolar mitotic figure (blue arrow, microscopic filed with 400X in haematoxylin and eosin stain), and (d) tumour cells showing strong intense cytoplasmic positivity for EMA (microscopic filed with 400X IHC).

Sarcomas will be Vimentin positive diffusely and SSTR2A negative. SFT will display staghorn vessels and positivity with CD34, STAT 6, BCL2 whereas negative for EMA and SSTR2A [12, 29, 40].

13.14 Papillary meningioma

They are categorised into CNS WHO grade 3. The tumour cells surround the thin walled blood vessels in a perivascular, pseudo rosette-like pattern. There is peritumoral oedema, bony destruction, hyperostosis reaction and rarely cyst formation [14]. A close genetic and molecular link is suggested between papillary and rhabdoid meningioma as few tumours display rhabdoid cytomorphology arranged in papillary architecture [62].

13.15 Rhabdoid meningioma

This subtype comes under CNS WHO grade 3. The tumour cells have typical rhabdoid morphology, which are large plump cells, with eccentrically placed round nuclei, open vesicular nuclear chromatin, prominent large nucleoli and hyaline paranuclear inclusions. Whorl formation is sometimes retained. Few tumour cells may have papillary features suggesting close association with papillary meningioma. These tumours have high mitotic activity and are aggressive in nature [14]. On immunohistochemistry, the tumour cells are EMA, PR, Vimentin positive. The inclusions are positive for cytokeratin. Characteristically, INI1 expression is retained [63].

14. Other rare variants of meningioma

14.1 Cystic meningioma

This variant accounts for 4–7% of meningiomas and is characterised by the presence of intratumoural or peritumoral cysts. The pathogenesis of cyst formation is tumour degeneration and necrosis which produces a macro–cavitation attributed to intracellular regressive process [64]. The content of the cyst may be CSF, xanthochromic fluid, clear fluid or haemorrhagic fluid [65].

There are four types of intracranial cystic meningiomas as per Nauta classification: [66].

i. Type 1–intratumoral cyst, present centrally, within the tumour

ii. Type 2–intratumoral cyst, present peripherally, surrounded by tumour

iii. Type 3–peritumoral cyst, present peripherally, adjacent to brain parenchyma

iv. Type 4–peritumoral cyst, present between tumour and brain parenchyma, cyst wall formed by arachnoid layer

14.2 Radiation induced meningioma (RIM)

This tumour occurs due to exposure to ionising radiation, with a long latent period of 2 to 63 years. These are multiple and aggressive. High grade RIM have increased

VEGH levels and mRNA overexpression [67]. These tumours have high MIB-1 labelling index of more than 10% due to increased proliferative activity and have a higher chance of recurrence within 1 year of resection [68].

14.3 Ossified meningioma

This variant comprises 1–5% and is located intraspinal or intracranial. It is a very slow growing tumour characterised by complete ossification/calcification of tumour foci. It is different from psammomatous meningioma, as viable meningothelial cells are present in the latter. It is considered as a subtype of grade 1 metaplastic meningioma as the pathogenesis postulated is the metaplastic change of arachnoid and interstitial cells [69, 70].

15. Squash cytology

Squash cytology is a simple, rapid and friendly technique for preliminary intraoperative diagnosis of CNS tumours/space occupying lesions. It helps to arrive at a reliable diagnosis on crush prep smears and gives guidance to the operating surgeon [71]. The cytological feature of meningioma seen on squash cytology include epithelioid cells with round to oval nuclei and delicate streaked cytoplasm. Sometimes, intranuclear pseudo inclusions are also noted. Meningothelial whorls/nests and psammoma bodies are highly characteristic. A major limitation observed is with tumours having abundant collagen and firm rubbery consistency, because adequate preparation of smears become difficult and challenging [12, 14].

Apart from the above described classical morphology, few subtypes of meningioma have additional characteristic specific features which provides a clue in their intra operative diagnosis:

- Chordoid meningioma–tumour cells are arranged as cords, have eosinophilic cytoplasm and embedded in an abundant myxoid rich background [72]

- Clear cell meningioma–spindled to polygonal cells having whorled and syncytial architecture, cells have bland nuclear chromatin and vacuolated cytoplasm [73]

- Rhabdoid meningioma–rhabdoid cells having eccentrically placed nuclei, vesicular chromatin, prominent nucleoli, dense eosinophilic cytoplasm and distinct cell borders. Cytoplasmic hyaline inclusions, pseudo nuclear inclusions, stout processes and increased mitotic activity may be identified [74]

- Papillary meningioma–papillary architecture seen on low power field [62]

- Anaplastic meningioma–increased atypical mitotic figures [40].

16. Conclusion

Meningioma is the most common tumour of CNS, seen most commonly in females at around 66 years of age, however rarely reported in children also. They can be asymptomatic or sometimes, symptomatic. Since the inception of WHO CNS blue books, with every edition, there has been an evolution in histopathological grading system of meningioma. The current WHO grading system has categorised meningioma into 3 grades. Grade 1 is the most common and has best prognosis. Grade 2 is intermediate and grade 3 is rare with worst prognosis. Various molecular and genetic alterations have been identified with novel diagnostic techniques. Immunohistochemistry helps to differentiate meningioma from other mimicking lesions and also helps to highlight entrapped glial tissue within the tumour foci. Squash cytology plays unique role in intra–operative diagnosis of the lesion with their characteristic morphology. Very rarely meningioma metastasize, however if present, lungs are the most common site.

17. Future aspects

Few more rare subtypes of meningiomas have been identified. These include oncocytic, mucinous, sclerosing, whorling–sclerosing, GFAP expressing, meningothelial rosettes and granulo-filamentous inclusion–bearing variants [75–77]. However, more studies and research is needed, to understand the same. Many treatment related (particularly immunotherapy) studies are being done, which is out of the purview of our chapter, as it focuses mainly on pathological aspects.

Acknowledgements

The authors wish to thank senior histopathology technical staff Mrs. Nazia and Mr. Rahul for excellent section cutting and staining.

Conflict of interest

The authors declare no conflict of interest.

Abbreviations

WHO	World Health Organisation
CNS	central nervous system
IHC	immunohistochemistry
NF2	neurofibromatosis type 2
VHL	Von Hippel Lindau
MEN1	multiple endocrine neoplasia type 1
YAP1	yes associated protein 1
AKT1	AKT serine/threonine kinase 1
PIK3CA	phosphatidyl inositol-4, 5-bisphosphate 3-kinase catalytic subunit alpha
TRAF7	TNF receptor associated factor 7
KLF4	kruppel like factor 4
SMO	protein smoothened
DNA	deoxyribo nucleic acid
TERT	telomerase reverse transcriptase

SMARCE1	SWI/SNF-related matrix-associated actin-dependent regulator of chromatin subfamily E member 1
CDKN2A/B	cyclin dependent kinase inhibitor 2A/B
FISH	fluorescence in situ hybridization
BAP1	BRCA1 associated protein 1
PBRM1	polybromo 1
RNA	ribo nucleic acid
H3 p.K28me3 (K27me3)	tri methylation of lysine 27 on histone H3
PI3K	phosphoinositide 3 kinases
POLR2A	RNA polymerase II subunit A
EMA	epithelial membrane antigen
SSTR2A	somatostatin receptor 2
ICD	international classification of diseases
MIB-1	E3 ubiquitin protein ligase
CEA	carcino embryonic antigen
GFAP	glial fibrillary acidic protein
NHERF1	Na+/H+ exchanger regulatory factor 1
PAS	periodic acid schiff
PR	progesterone receptor
CK AE1/AE3	cytokeratin AE1/AE3
STAT6	signal transducer and activator of transcription 6
SFT	solitary fibrous tumour
HMB45	human melanoma black 45
CD34	cluster of differentiation 34
BCL2	B cell lymphoma 2
INI1	integrase interactor 1
CSF	cerebro spinal fluid
RIM	radiation induced meningioma
VEGF	vascular endothelial growth factor
mRNA	messenger ribonucleic acid

Author details

Amit Kumar Chowhan and Mousmi Agrawal*
Department of Pathology and Lab Medicine, All India Institute of Medical Sciences (AIIMS), Raipur, Chhattisgarh, India

*Address all correspondence to: mousmiasrc@gmail.com

References

[1] Ostrom QT, Cioffi G, Gittleman H, Patil N, Waite K, Kruchko C, et al. CBTRUS statistical report: Primary brain and other central nervous system Tumors diagnosed in the United States in 2012-2016. Neuro-Oncology. 2019;**21**(5):v1-v100

[2] Wiemels J, Wrensch M, Claus EB. Epidemiology and etiology of meningioma. Journal of Neuro-Oncolology. 2010;**99**(3):307-314

[3] Toland A, Huntoon K, Dahiya SM. Meningioma: A pathology perspective. Neurosurgery. 2021;**89**(1):11-21

[4] Cushing H. The meningiomas (dural endotheliomas): Their source and favored seats of origin (cavendish lecture). Brain. 1922;**45**:282-316

[5] Barthelemy EJ, Sarkiss CA, Lee J, Shrivastava RK. The historical origin of the term "meningioma" and the rise of nationalistic neurosurgery. Journal of Neurosurgery. 2016;**125**(5):1283-1290

[6] Lee JH. Meningiomas: Diagnosis, treatment, and outcome. American Journal of Neuroradiology. 2009;**30**(10):E157

[7] Cohen AR. William Macewen and the first documented successful resection of a brain tumor. Child's Nervous System. 2023;**39**:3019-3024. DOI: 10.1007/s00381-023-05825-3

[8] Louis DN, Ohgaki H, Wiestler OD, Cavenee WK, Burger PC, Jouvet A, et al. The 2007 WHO classification of tumours of the central nervous system. Acta Neuropathologica. 2007;**114**(2):97-109

[9] Ogasawara C, Philbrick BD, Adamson DC. Meningioma: A review of epidemiology, pathology, diagnosis, treatment, and future directions. Biomedicine. 2021;**9**(3):319

[10] Johnson MD, Abu-Farsakh S. Clinicopathologic features of incidental meningiomas: A review of the literature and the University of Rochester Autopsy experience. Clinical Neuropathology. 2019;**38**:118-121

[11] Varlotto J, Flickinger J, Pavelic MT, Specht CS, Sheehan JM, Timek DT, et al. Distinguishing grade I meningioma from higher grade meningiomas without biopsy. Oncotarget. 2015;**6**(35):38421-38428

[12] Backer-Grondahl T, Moen BH, Torp SH. The histopathological spectrum of human meningiomas. International Journal of Clinical and Experimental Pathology. 2012;**5**(3):231-242

[13] Clark VE, Erson-Omay EZ, Serin A, Yin J, Cotney J, Ozduman K, et al. Genomic analysis of non-NF2 meningiomas reveals mutations in TRAF7, KLF4, AKT1, and SMO. Science. 2013;**339**(6123):1077-1080

[14] Louis DN, Sahm F, Perry A, et al. Meningioma. In: WHO Classification of Tumours Editorial Board. Central Nervous System Tumours. Lyon (France): International Agency for Research on Cancer; 2021. (WHO classification of tumours series, 5th ed.; vol. 6). Available from: https://tumourclassification.iarc.who.int/chapters/45

[15] Zhang H, Ma L, Shu C, Dong LQ, Ma YQ, Zhou Y. Spinal clear cell meningiomas: Clinical features and factors predicting recurrence. World Neurosurgery. 2020;**134**:e1062-e1076

[16] Rushing EJ, Bouffard JP, McCall S, Olsen C, Mena H, Sandberg GD, et al. Primary extracranial meningiomas: An analysis of 146 cases. Head and Neck Pathology. 2009;**3**(2):116-130

[17] Moran CA, Hochholzer L, Rush W, Koss MN. Primary intrapulmonary meningiomas. A clinicopathologic and immunohistochemical study of ten cases. Cancer. 1996;**78**(11):2328-2333

[18] Deshmukh SD, Rokade VV, Pathak GS, Nemade SV, Ashturkar AV. Primary extra-cranial meningioma in the right submandibular region of an 18-year-old woman: A case report. Journal of Medical Case Reports. 2011;**5**:271

[19] Mogi A, Hirato J, Kosaka T, Yamaki E, Kuwano H. Primary mediastinal atypical meningioma: Report of a case and literature review. World Journal of Surgical Oncology. 2012;**10**:17

[20] Sievers P, Chiang J, Schrimpf D, Stichel D, Paramasivam N, Sill M, et al. YAP1-fusions in pediatric NF2-wildtype meningioma. Acta Neuropathologica. 2020;**139**(1):215-218

[21] Brastianos PK, Horowitz PM, Santagata S, Jones RT, McKenna A, Getz G, et al. Genomic sequencing of meningiomas identifies oncogenic SMO and AKT1 mutations. Nature Genetics. 2013;**45**(3):285-289

[22] Louis DN, Perry A, Wesseling P, Brat DJ, Cree IA, Figarella-Branger D, et al. The 2021 WHO classification of Tumors of the central nervous system: A summary. Neuro-Oncology. 2021;**23**(8):1231-1251

[23] Sahm F, Bissel J, Koelsche C, Schweizer L, Capper D, Reuss D, et al. AKT1E17K mutations cluster with meningothelial and transitional meningiomas and can be detected by SFRP1 immunohistochemistry. Acta Neuropathologica. 2013;**126**(5):757-762

[24] Fountain DM, Smith MJ, O'Leary C, Pathmanaban ON, Roncaroli F, Bobola N, et al. The spatial phenotype of genotypically distinct meningiomas demonstrate potential implications of the embryology of the meninges. Oncogene. 2021;**40**(5):875-884

[25] Abedalthagafi MS, Merrill PH, Bi WL, Jones RT, Listewnik ML, Ramkissoon SH, et al. Angiomatous meningiomas have a distinct genetic profile with multiple chromosomal polysomies including polysomy of chromosome 5. Oncotarget. 2014;**5**(21):10596-10606

[26] Sievers P, Stichel D, Hielscher T, Schrimpf D, Reinhardt A, Wefers AK, et al. Chordoid meningiomas can be sub-stratified into prognostically distinct DNA methylation classes and are enriched for heterozygous deletions of chromosomal arm 2p. Acta Neuropathologica. 2018;**136**(6):975-978

[27] Tauziede-Espariat A, Parfait B, Besnard A, Lacombe J, Pallud J, Tazi S, et al. Loss of SMARCE1 expression is a specific diagnostic marker of clear cell meningioma: A comprehensive immunophenotypical and molecular analysis. Brain Pathology. 2018;**28**(4):466-474

[28] Goutagny S, Nault JC, Mallet M, Henin D, Rossi JZ, Kalamarides M. High incidence of activating TERT promoter mutations in meningiomas undergoing malignant progression. Brain Pathology. 2014;**24**(2):184-189

[29] Bostrom J, Meyer-Puttlitz B, Wolter M, Blaschke B, Weber RG, Lichter P, et al. Alterations of the tumor suppressor genes CDKN2A

(p16(INK4a)), p14(ARF), CDKN2B (p15(INK4b)), and CDKN2C (p18(INK4c)) in atypical and anaplastic meningiomas. The Americal Journal of Pathology. 2001;**159**(2):661-669

[30] Katz LM, Hielscher T, Liechty B, Silverman J, Zagzag D, Sen R, et al. Loss of histone H3K27me3 identifies a subset of meningiomas with increased risk of recurrence. Acta Neuropathologica. 2018;**135**(6):955-963

[31] Sahm F, Toprak UH, Hubschmann D, Kleinheinz K, Buchhalter I, Sill M, et al. Meningiomas induced by low-dose radiation carry structural variants of NF2 and a distinct mutational signature. Acta Neuropathologica. 2017;**134**(1):155-158

[32] Brenner AV, Sugiyama H, Preston DL, Sakata R, French B, Sadakane A, et al. Radiation risk of central nervous system tumors in the life span study of atomic bomb survivors, 1958-2009. European Journal of Epidemiology. 2020;**35**(6):591-600

[33] Claus EB, Calvocoressi L, Bondy ML, Wrensch M, Wiemels JL, Schildkraut JM. Exogenous hormone use, reproductive factors, and risk of intracranial meningioma in females. Journal of Neurosurgery. 2013;**118**(3):649-656

[34] Niedermaier T, Behrens G, Schmid D, Schlecht I, Fischer B, Leitzmann MF. Body mass index, physical activity, and risk of adult meningioma and glioma: A meta-analysis. Neurology. 2015;**85**(15):1342-1350

[35] Kane AJ, Sughrue ME, Rutkowski MJ, Shangari G, Fang S, McDermott MW, et al. Anatomic location is a risk factor for atypical and malignant meningiomas. Cancer. 2011;**117**(6):1272-1278

[36] Du Z, Santagata S. Uncovering the links between systemic hormones and oncogenic signaling in the pathogenesis of meningioma. Annals of Oncology. 2018;**29**(3):537-540

[37] Christiaans I, Kenter SB, Brink HC, van Os TA, Baas F, van den Munckhof P, et al. Germline SMARCB1 mutation and somatic NF2 mutations in familial multiple meningiomas. Journal of Medical Genetics. 2011;**48**(2):93-97

[38] Maiuri F, Mariniello G, Somma T, Guadagno E, Corvino S, Pagano S, et al. Meningiomas in premenopausal women: Role of the hormone related conditions. Frontiers in Oncology. 2020;**10**:556701

[39] Wang PF, Ji WJ, Zhang XH, Li SW, Yan CX. Allergy reduces the risk of meningioma: A meta-analysis. Scientific Reports. 2017;**7**:40333

[40] Buttrick S, Shah AH, Komotar RJ, Ivan ME. Management of Atypical and Anaplastic Meningiomas. Neurosurgery Clinics of North America. 2016;**27**(2):239-247

[41] Buerki RA, Horbinski CM, Kruser T, Horowitz PM, James CD, Lukas RV. An overview of meningiomas. Future Oncology. 2018;**14**(21):2161-2177

[42] Elwatidy SM, Albakr AA, Al Towim AA, Malik SH. Tumors of the lateral and third ventricle: Surgical management and outcome analysis in 42 cases. Neurosciences (Riyadh). 2017;**22**(4):274-281

[43] Ciftdemir M, Kaya M, Selcuk E, Yalniz E. Tumors of the spine. World Journal of Orthopedics. 2016;**7**(2):109-116

[44] Vuong HG, Ngo TNM, Dunn IF. Incidence, risk factors, and prognosis of meningiomas with distant metastases at presentation. Neuro-oncology. Advances. 2021;**3**(1):vdab084

[45] Kleihues P, Burger PC, Scheithauer BW. The new WHO classification of brain tumours. Brain Pathology. 1993;**3**(3):255-268

[46] Scheithauer BW. Development of the WHO classification of tumors of the central nervous system: A historical perspective. Brain Pathology. 2009;**19**(4):551-564

[47] Louis DN, Budka H, Von Deimling A. Meningiomas. In: Kleihues P, Cavenee WK, editors. World Health Organization Classification of Tumours. Pathology and Genetics of Tumours of the Nervous System. Lyon, France: IARC Press; 1993. pp. 134-141

[48] Kleihues P, Louis DN, Scheithauer BW, Rorke LB, Reifenberger G, Burger PC, et al. The WHO classification of tumors of the nervous system. Journal of Neuropathology and Experimental Neurology. 2002;**61**(3):215-225

[49] Perry A, Scheithauer BW, Stafford SL, Lohse CM, Wollan PC. "Malignancy" in meningiomas: A clinicopathologic study of 116 patients, with grading implications. Cancer. 1999;**85**:2046-2056

[50] Perry A, Stafford SL, Scheithauer BW, Suman VJ, Lohse CM. Meningioma grading: An analysis of histologic parameters. The American Journal of Surgical Pathology. 1997;**21**:1455-1465

[51] Perry A, Louis DN, Scheithauer BW, Budka H, von Diemling A. Meningiomas. In: Louis DN, Ohgaki H, Wiestler OD, et al., editors. World Health Organization Classification of Tumours of the Central Nervous System. 4th ed. Lyon: IARC; 2007. pp. 164-172

[52] Perry A, Chicoine MR, Filiput E, Miller JP, Cross DT. Clinicopathologic assessment and grading of embolized meningiomas: A correlative study of 64 patients. Cancer. 2001;**92**:701-711

[53] Chkheidze R, Cimino PJ, Hatanpaa KJ, White CL, Ferreira M, Piccirillo SGM, et al. Distinct expression patterns of carbonic anhydrase IX in clear cell, microcystic, and angiomatous meningiomas. Journal of Neuropathholology and Experimental Neurology. 2019;**78**(12):1081-1088

[54] Louis DN, Hamilton AJ, Sobel RA, Ojemann RG. Pseudopsammomatous meningioma with elevated serum carcinoembryonic antigen: A true secretory meningioma. Case report. Journal of Neurosurgery. 1991;**74**(1):129-132

[55] Lal A, Dahiya S, Gonzales M, Hiniker A, Prayson R, Kleinschmidt-DeMasters BK, et al. IgG4 overexpression is rare in meningiomas with a prominent inflammatory component: A review of 16 cases. Brain Pathology. 2014;**24**(4):352-359

[56] Aghi MK, Carter BS, Cosgrove GR, Ojemann RG, Amin-Hanjani S, Martuza RL, et al. Long-term recurrence rates of atypical meningiomas after gross total resection with or without postoperative adjuvant radiation. Neurosurgery. 2009;**64**(1):56-60

[57] Gabeau-Lacet D, Aghi M, Betensky RA, Barker FG, Loeffler JS, Louis DN. Bone involvement predicts poor outcome in atypical meningioma. Journal of Neurosurgery. 2009;**111**(3):464-471

[58] Couce ME, Aker FV, Scheithauer BW. Chordoid meningioma: A clinicopathologic study of 42 cases. The American Journal of Surgical Pathology. 2000;**24**(7):899-905

[59] Choy W, Ampie L, Lamano JB, Kesavabhotla K, Mao Q, Parsa AT, et al. Predictors of recurrence in the management of chordoid meningioma. Journal of Neuro-Oncology. 2016;**126**(1):107-116

[60] Georgescu MM, Olar A, Mobley BC, Faust PL, Raisanen JM. Epithelial differentiation with microlumen formation in meningioma: Diagnostic utility of NHERF1/EBP50 immunohistochemistry. Oncotarget. 2018;**9**(47):28652-28665

[61] Kepes JJ, Chen WY, Connors MH, Vogel FS. "chordoid" meningeal tumors in young individuals with peritumoral lymphoplasmacellular infiltrates causing systemic manifestations of the Castleman syndrome. A report of seven cases. Cancer. 1988;**62**(2):391-406

[62] Wu YT, Ho JT, Lin YJ, Lin JW. Rhabdoid papillary meningioma: A clinicopathologic case series study. Neuropathology. 2011;**31**(6):599-605

[63] Perry A, Fuller CE, Judkins AR, Dehner LP, Biegel JA. INI1 expression is retained in composite rhabdoid tumors, including rhabdoid meningiomas. Modern Pathology. 2005;**18**(7):951-958

[64] Wang P, Han S, Liu N, Yu C, Qi X, Zhu M, et al. Peritumoral cystic meningioma: A report of two cases and review of the literature. Experimental and Therapeutic Medicine. 2016;**11**(3):904-908

[65] el-Fiki M, el-Henawy Y, Abdel-Rahman N. Cystic meningioma. Acta Neurochirurgica. 1996;**138**(7):811-817

[66] Nauta HJ, Tucker WS, Horsey WJ, Bilbao JM, Gonsalves C. Xanthochromic cysts associated with meningioma. Journal of Neurology, Neurosurgery & Psychiatry. 1979;**42**(6):529-535

[67] Mansouri A, Badhiwala J, Mansouri S, Zadeh G. The evolving role of radiosurgery in the management of radiation-induced meningiomas: A review of current advances and future directions. BioMedical Research International. 2014;**2014**:107526

[68] Goto Y, Yamada S, Yamada SM, Nakaguchi H, Hoya K, Murakami M, et al. Radiation-induced meningiomas in multiple regions, showing rapid recurrence and a high MIB 1 labeling index: A case report and review of the literature. World Journal of Surgical Oncology. 2014;**12**:123

[69] Murakami T, Tanishima S, Takeda C, Kato S, Nagashima H. Ossified metaplastic spinal meningioma without Psammomatous calcification: A case report. Yonago Acta Medica. 2019;**62**(2):232-235

[70] Taha MM, Alawamry A, Abdel-Aziz HR. Ossified spinal meningioma: A case report and a review of the literature. The Surgery Journal. 2019;**5**(4):e137-e141

[71] Shri LS. Meningiomas: A clinicopathological study. International Journal of Medical Research and Health Sciences. 2015;**4**(4):827-831

[72] Yagi C, Yamamuro S, Ozawa Y, Yoshimura S, Sumi K, Yoshino A. A case of tuberculum sellae chordoid meningioma treated via extended endoscopic endonasal trans-sphenoidal surgery. NMC Case Report Journal. 2020;**7**(2):53-56

[73] Imlay SP, Snider TE, Raab SS. Clear-cell meningioma: Diagnosis by fine-needle aspiration biopsy. Diagnostic Cytopathology. 1998;**18**(2):131-136

[74] Bansal M, Pathak VP, Kishore S, Bansal KK. Rhabdoid meningioma: Rapid intraoperative diagnosis on squash smears. Diagnostic Cytopathology. 2010;**38**(8):594-596

[75] Gallina P, Buccoliero AM, Mariotti F, Mennonna P, Di Lorenzo N. Oncocytic meningiomas: Cases with benign histopathological features and a favorable clinical course. Journal of Neurosurgery. 2006;**105**(5):736-738

[76] Haberler C, Jarius C, Lang S, Rossler K, Gruber A, Hainfellner JA, et al. Fibrous meningeal tumours with extensive non-calcifying collagenous whorls and glial fibrillary acidic protein expression: The whorling-sclerosing variant of meningioma. Neuropathology and Applied Neurobiology. 2002;**28**(1):42-47

[77] Berho M, Suster S. Mucinous meningioma. Report of an unusual variant of meningioma that may mimic metastatic mucin-producing carcinoma. The American Journal of Surgical Pathology. 1994;**18**(1):100-106